KU-186-366

Contents

Foreword

The Health Education Authority must be congratulated on publication of the proceedings of this conference which emphasised the need for a comprehensive policy for sexual health promotion and highlighted some of the opportunities and challenges in implementing *The Health of the Nation* in a GUM clinic setting. Public health doctors have roles in planning and developing strategies for sexual health promotion, and for purchasing sexual health services. We are concerned that health promotion strategies are successful in adapting national targets for local situations, and that services are effective.

If we are to achieve *The Health of the Nation* targets on sexual health it is important that every opportunity is taken to deliver a more broad-based sexual health and reproductive health care service. One of the recommendations from this conference is for closer collaboration between the disciplines involved in family planning and sexually transmitted diseases. The Faculty of Public Health Medicine will be taking this forward by holding a consensus workshop on sexual health promotion and service provision, in collaboration with the Faculty of Family Planning and Reproductive Health Care of the Royal College of Obstetricians and Gynaecologists and the Medical Society for the Study of Venereal Diseases.

Michael O'Brien

J. M. O'Brien
President, Faculty of Public Health Medicine, Royal College of Physicians

Contributors

Introduction. Dr Jayshree Pillaye, Senior Medical Officer, Health Education Authority.
1. Professor Max Elstein, Department of Obstetrics and Gynaecology, University Hospital of South Manchester.
    Dr Yvonne Steadman, Consultant, Worcester Community Trust, formerly Withington Hospital, Manchester.
2. Dr Jayshree Pillay, Senior Medical Officer, Health Education Authority.
3. Mr Peter Greenhouse, Consultant, Sexual Health Clinic, Ipswich.
4. Dr Fiona Boag, Consultant, John Hunter Clinic, Kensington and Chelsea, London.
5. Tim Rhodes, Researcher, Centre for Research on Drugs and Behaviour.
6. Shivanda Khan, Director, the NAZ Project – an HIV/AIDS education prevention and support service for South Asian, Turkish, Irani and Arab communities.
7. Jef Jones, Education Section Manager, Terrence Higgins Trust, London.
8. Elspeth Gould, Senior Health Adviser, Genitourinary Medicine Clinic, Newcastle General Hospital, Newcastle.
9. Mohammed Rajabali, CRUSAID.
10. Veronica Poon, Clinical Nurse Specialist, Florey Unit, Royal Berkshire Hospital, Reading.
11. Rochelle Bloch, Senior Commissioning Manager for HIV/AIDS and Substance Abuse.
    Anthony Worth, HIV Prevention Coordinator, Ealing, Hammersmith and Hounslow Health Agency, London.
12. Dr George Kinghorn, Clinical Director, Department of Genitourinary Medicine, Royal Hallamshire Hospital, Sheffield.

Introduction

Dr Jayshree Pillaye

A conference on Sexual Health Promotion in Genitourinary Medicine Clinics was held in London on 4 March 1994. The main aim of the meeting was to explore the opportunities and challenges for wider sexual health promotion in a genitourinary medicine (GUM) clinic setting. The programme was designed to emphasise the need for a broad-based approach to sexual health service provision; taking into account health professional variability in terms of skills and training, the widely differing needs of patients, and the different models of service provision in the country. GUM clinics are staffed by a multidisciplinary team. This presents challenges in defining roles and responsibilities to optimise patient care. Patient variability in terms of culture, individual attitudes and value systems, sexual orientation and risk factors are further challenges to maximising opportunistic sexual health promotion in a GUM clinic setting.

Sexual health is one of the key areas mentioned in *The Health of the Nation*[1]. Sexually transmitted diseases (STDs) including HIV infection and hepatitis B, unplanned pregnancies and drug misuse are major public health issues nationally and internationally. *The Health of the Nation* sets out objectives for sexual health, to:

- reduce the incidence of HIV infection;
- reduce the incidence of other STDs;
- develop further and strengthen monitoring and surveillance;
- provide effective services for diagnosis and treatment of HIV and other STDs;
- reduce the number of unwanted pregnancies;
- ensure the provision of effective family planning services for those people who want them.

The targets are to reduce:

- the incidence of gonorrhoea among men and women aged 15–64 by at least 20% by 1995 (from 61 new cases per 100,000 population in 1990 to no more than 49 new cases per 100,000);
- the rate of conceptions amongst the under-16s by at least 50% by the year 2000 (from 9.5 per 1000 girls aged 13–15 in 1989 to no more than 4.8);
- the percentage of injecting drug misusers who report sharing injecting equipment in

1

the previous four weeks by at least 50% by 1997, and by at least a further 50% by the year 2000 (from 20% in 1990 to no more than 10% by 1997 and no more than 5% by the year 2000). '

GUM clinics therefore have a crucial role in the health of the nation because they have a captive audience for wider sexual health promotion.

The most important barriers to health promotion in the control of STDs and HIV infection area[2] are:

- Low perception of risk.
- Negative attitudes towards the use of condoms (including beliefs about ineffectiveness and unacceptability).
- Alcohol and illicit drug use.
- Absence of social support for behavioural change.

What do we mean by sexual health?

In 1974 the World Health Organization (WHO) defined sexual health as 'the integration of the physical, emotional, intellectual and social aspects of sexual being, in ways that are enriching and that enhance communication and love'.

This definition is rather utopian. Sexual health is an important aspect of general health, but the definition continues to be elusive. It is difficult to include everyone's concept of sexuality in one definition. Sexual health is influenced by a variety of factors (Fig I.1) that affect general health including:

- Biological and physiological function.
- Cultural factors including religion and sub-cultures.
- Social and personal value systems – i.e. what is regarded as good or bad, or appropriate and inappropriate.
- Biological sex.
- Sexual orientation.
- Body image.
- Environmental factors/situations.
- Gender power.
- Interpersonal skills.
- Legal and moral sanctions.
- Media.

Sexual health encompasses both the physical and psychological aspects of sexuality, and promotes general health. It includes emotional and physical pleasure without the risk of acquiring or transmitting infection, and with the ability to control fertility. Healthy sexuality has inherent rights and obligations; the right of a person to decide for him/herself how they wish to express themselves as a sexual being, but with the obligation not to harm others. The right to enjoy their sexuality free from fear, shame or guilt, but with the obligation not to oppress or coerce. Healthy sexuality promotes self-esteem, and positive self-esteem promotes sexual health.

Some prerequisites for health professionals to promote sexual health include:
- An ability to recognise sexual problems.
- To be comfortable when discussing sexuality with people of either gender, and irrespective of sexual orientation.
- To be aware of culture-specific sexual practices which should be addressed appropriately and sensitively.
- To be able to address opportunistically a range of preventive issues related to

sexual health (education, information and screening).
- To have the competency to make appropriate referrals.

Most of these issues were addressed by the speakers and by members of the audience in the discussion that followed.

First morning session

This was chaired by Dr Meg Weir, from the Department of Health and covered the need, opportunities and barriers to providing an opportunistic/integrated contraceptive service for women attending GUM clinics. The emphasis was on the importance of organisational and professional commitment necessary to merge the skills, and knowledge base of family planning and STD services. It also highlights the role of the different professional bodies and organisations (Faculty of Family Planning and Reproductive Health Care, Faculty of Public Health Medicine and the Medical Society for the Study of Venereal Disease) in working together. The role of public education and information was also stressed, and that this should include a unified preventive

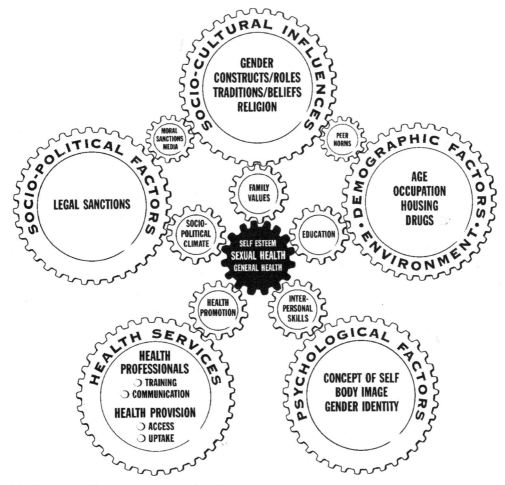

Fig I.1: Factors influencing sexual health

approach towards both STD and unintended pregnancies. The overlapping needs of women provide a unique opportunity to deliver a more broad-based reproductive health care.

Prof. Max Elstein and Dr Yvonne Steadman (Chapter 1) emphasised that the merging of these two disciplines was especially important for young people. Prof. Elstein outlined the differences in the two disciplines of family planning and STDs in this country. Dr Steadman showed the needs of young women attending family planning and GUM clinics overlap; and stressed the need for agreed protocols for referrals, and the importance of training of family planning and GUM personnel. In South Manchester this has been achieved by sharing personnel. Nursing staff work in family planning and GUM clinics, and all family planning doctors can work in GUM clinics for six months.

The preliminary results from a short patient survey of sexual health promotion in GUM clinics are discussed in Chapter 2. The aim of the survey was to gauge patients' perception of their clinic visit, and whether they had information and services for wider sexual health promotion. The report covered patients' views on posters, leaflets, discussion of safer sex – including the use of drugs and alcohol – contraception, cervical smears, perception of visit and attitudes to stigma and confidentiality. Dr Pillaye concluded that the patients interviewed wished to receive sexual health promotion, including contraceptive advice at their GUM clinic visit. However, there still appeared some stigma attached to attending a GUM clinic, and clinic attenders did not wish others (including their general practitioner) to know about their visit.

Mr Peter Greenhouse (Chapter 3) explored sexual health services under one roof. He remarked that there is a split in the provision of sexual health care, not just between the different specialties of family planning, gynaecology and what used to be called venereology, but between the way the services are advertised or promoted. He claimed that this was damaging both to the health promotional message and to the provision of services; and showed that the principal shift in emphasis should be away from the clinic attended by individuals when there is something really wrong, to a clinic that is attended to check that an individual is healthy. He declared that he would like to see sexual health under one roof, and that the public health arguments for a unified health care for women are now overwhelming. He concluded that, perhaps the only way that this will advance is when women's health is both planned and provided by women for women.

Dr Fiona Boag (Chapter 4) discussed the women only session held within the GUM clinic. This session provided an integrated health care, including HIV, sexually transmitted infections, and family planning. There were twice the number of new patients coming to the women's clinic as to the John Hunter GUM clinic. During the first year, approximately 60% of the new HIV positive women in the unit came through the women's clinic. Family planning services were brought on board because of a high risk of unwanted pregnancy in the clinic attenders.

Second morning session

This was chaired by Peter Weatherburn from Project SIGMA and covered sexual health promotion beyond contraception. This highlights the comprehensive and multidisciplinary nature of sexual health provision services. When a patient attends a GUM clinic, health professionals may find it easier to treat an infection, than to discuss aspects of sexuality, sexual partners and drug use. However, these are important issues that GUM clinics have to take on board if they are to maintain a role in sexual health promotion. The speakers expressed concerns about communication between health professionals and patients, especially with patients from minority cultures.

Tim Rhodes (Chapter 5) presented findings on the sexual behaviour of drug injectors – recruited as part of an ongoing WHO funded study. He explained that epidemiological data showed that the majority of drug injectors are sexually active and the majority are at risk of STDs because they may prioritise safer drug use to safer sex. He pointed out that many drug injectors and drug users are not accessing sexual health and GUM services, and when they do so, or when they do access drug-related services, they tend to prioritise things other than sexual health. He concluded that drug injectors are going to be less likely to change their sexual behaviour if they do not see unsafe sex as risky.

Shivananda Khan (Chapter 6) discussed sexual health issues with regard to minority ethnic communities. He referred to the paucity of data in this area, and emphasised that the minority communities were not homogenous groups, and challenged some of the stereotypes that abound about minority ethnic communities, especially in relation to sex. A major concern of minority ethnic communities in this country was racism. He also discussed the different constructions of South Asian cultures in relation to terminology, and concepts of shame and guilt.

Jef Jones (Chapter 7) discussed sexuality awareness. According to Jones it is bound up with our gender – and the genders of the people to whom we also may be sexually attracted. He pointed out that people's sexuality is related to their actual sexual practices, cultures, fantasies and to sexual images. The task of education, of diagnosis, treatment and of care requires that an objective and uninvolved perspective be maintained. In the clinics where staff are encouraged to go through that process in training, in consultancy, in support and supervision, patients are not just equally treated, but their sexuality is dignified and celebrated.

Elspeth Gould (Chapter 8) discussed contact tracing and partner notification. She referred to patient referral and provider referral as complementary aspects of partner notification. Whether or not partners are found to have infection, the process of partner notification targets the health promotion skills and activities of the clinic team to people who are known to have been at risk of STDs. The greater proportion of referral work is done by the patients themselves – with a lot of backup from the health care workers. In a seven-year period since HIV was first known in Newcastle, the vast majority of partner notification was patient referral, and 21.9% of their newly diagnosed HIV positive patients attended as a result of partner notification.

Afternoon session

This was chaired by Isobel Allen, of the Policy Studies Institute, and looked at the role consumers, providers and purchasers play in sexual health promotion in GUM clinics. Health care services, including GUM and sexual health services have and continue to undergo change. The purchaser–provider split, audit and quality control and monitoring may result in a more effective service provision, and should provide better models for sexual health promotion. This session, however, raised more questions, than provided answers.

Mohammed Rajabali (Chapter 9) discussed some of the issues facing clients when they visit a GUM clinic. He mentioned the anxiety, fear and shame experienced by patients, and that the attitude of the nurses, doctors and social workers is extremely important on the first visit. He spoke about the difficulties young gay men have, and all the associated anxieties of being HIV-positive. He also addressed practical issues like appointments, waiting time, continuity of care and crèche facilities. He concluded that a discussion on lifestyles was paramount, and that patients should be presented with choices.

Veronica Poon (Chapter 10) discussed the role and responsibility of a clinical nurse specialist in the GUM clinic, and how this may vary from clinic to clinic. She remarked that many qualified nurses have little or no knowledge about the working of a GUM clinic. The clinical nurse specialist, therefore, provides information about the services of a department of GUM so that nurses have a better understanding of the service, are able to explain to their clients the facilities available and encourage them to use its services.

Rochelle Bloch and Anthony Worth (Chapter 11) discussed sexual health promotion in a GUM clinic from a purchaser's perspective. They emphasised the role of health promotion in providing service development support to GUM clinics, and that it was important to set structures which meet service users' requirements as well as purchasing requirements. Potential problems with GUM services could be avoided if there was collaborative planning and provision of models of good practice. Purchasers should be cognisant of the costs involved in treating some of the sequelae of STDs, and it is important that people come to GUM clinics with asymptomatic diseases so that long-term sequelae and secondary infection can be prevented.

Dr George Kinghorn (Chapter 12) spoke from a clinical director's perspective. He stressed that GUM clinics have as their major service objectives the diagnosis, treatment and control of sexually transmitted diseases. He pointed out that success in these objectives necessitated early patient presentation, screening of at-risk individuals, reliable laboratory diagnostic procedures, effective treatment and contact tracing. He thought it was difficult to get some health professionals involved in HIV/AIDS prevention and treatment to understand the association with other STDs and sexual health problems. He found that the funding of GUM services (related to the numbers of new patients and the total of clinic attenders) is based upon the number of ill patients seen and that there is little or no reward for disease prevention. An issue often raised is the lack of hard data on the effectiveness of sexual health promotion to persuade cynical purchasers. Kinghorn concluded by posing a question about sexual health promotion – not 'Can we afford it?', but 'Can we afford not to?'.

References

1. Department of Health (1992). *The Health of the Nation: A Strategy for Health in England*, Cm 1986. HMSO.
2. Hankins, C. (1990). Prevention of sexually transmitted diseases. Whose responsibility? What message? *Can. Med. Assoc. J.* **143**(8), 717–18.

1 Sexual health promotion and family planning in genitourinary medicine clinics

Prof. Max Elstein and Dr Yvonne Steadman

Family planning and sexually transmitted diseases – Max Elstein

Introduction

We are going to present a duet to you, with me providing the beginning and the after-end, and my colleague Yvonne Steadman discussing the needs of both family planning and STD patients, as she works in both these areas.

We hope to highlight the issues and implications of sexual activity, particularly for youngsters. These are STDs and unplanned pregnancies. There are some similarities and differences, and I would like to identify those, and talk about the need in the community and point a way forward.

The Health of the Nation is a way forward. I aim to highlight the particular issue of 'service provision', and the whole issue of unplanned pregnancies and STDs.

Unplanned pregnancies and STDs

There are two disciplines that deal with these issues, and these have to come together. There are differences and similarities that I would like to bring to your attention.

Women really 'carry the can – or the baby'. STDs in women are far more severe, far more debilitating and cause ill health to a far greater extent than in men. The difficulty is that they are asymptomatic, and we now see younger age people; and usually, in my clinic, I see the odd case of youngsters in their early 20s who are 'pelvic cripples'. I have to decide on radical management of them. We also have had an exacerbation of treatment of women for infertility, and most of these women in their 30s who have infertility are often a throwback to what happened to them when they were young. This is sad because, with good advice, good service and good education many of these problems are preventable.

What are the differences in these two issues in people? First of all, the prevalence of fertility is much higher than the prevalence of people who are at risk of becoming infected. But the difficulty is that each time an individual has sexual relationships, even without ejaculation, there is a risk of a sexually transmitted disease. Whereas, every time that a couple have intercourse, the risk of pregnancy is not as high as some people believe, it is about 20% at most – so the risk is lower. You have got to have frequent intercourse to become pregnant. But, getting an STD depends on whom you have the relationship with, and on how many people you have sexual relationships with.

So, what are the differences in the two disciplines and the backgrounds dealing with these two issues?.[1]

There are a number of issues, each of which has a difference in the background of STDs (bacteriology) and family planning (contraceptive technology). Fortunately, we are moving closer together and I think this is part and parcel of the message I wish to bring to you.

What advances have there been? We have had advances in the diagnosis, but not all these advances are available across the country. Also, we have had advances in better and more specific antibiotics (and fewer side-effects from these antibiotics), but essentially the thrust of the advances in family planning has been different. These are based on endocrinology, on more sophisticated hormonal manipulations, and on the quality of service provision.

The counselling process in STD is usually related to the way it presents. Whereas, with family planning the ethos is one of accepting, non-judgemental and indicating choices. There is a case to be made, and a strong case to be made, for that attitude to enter into some STD services. I know STD services have improved remarkably in the last decade, but that needs to be more widely based. For example, the focus of STD was primarily a male issue, at least a decade ago. Fortunately, there is a change, and we would hear about that change in these contributions.

Family planning has been primarily run by lady doctors, providing a very effective service. There needs to be more involvement of both sexes in providing family planning services in Britain. Here, we are in fact, in advance of many other countries in the world.

So there are differences, and we should bring these together and have a greater commonality of approach. This is possibly 'old hat' to you all, but, really, we are facing a crisis in the unplanned pregnancy rate and the crisis is affecting the young (in spite of wide availability of contraception), and in spite of all the messages, it is affecting the youngsters more and more.

The needs of young women attending family planning and GUM clinics – Yvonne Steadman

I work in both areas: family planning and GUM, and these are areas which are particularly close to my heart, because not a day goes by when somebody will not be seen, in one of the other clinics, who is in real need of counselling about all aspects of sexual health. I think we must get away from this division in the service between family planning, whether it is delivered by family planning doctors or by GPs, and genitourinary medicine. As already discussed, the division is a historical one – the time has now come for the services to collaborate and liaise with each other. One of the main problems is that we do not at the moment have a method that protects effectively against pregnancy and also protects effectively against sexually transmitted infections. Of course, the pill is the most effective method of preventing a pregnancy and is most commonly used, whereas the method that protects against infections is the condom. So there has been that divergence which has been perpetuated by the fact that there is no ideal method which meets both needs. But, perhaps what we have to contend with is the overlapping clinical need. I think it is very important to recognise that the groups of patients we see in our different clinics are the same groups of women. There is not just a group of women who go along to family planning clinics, and yet another group who go along to STD clinics. They are the same women, and I think it is very important that we remember that. Like it or not, our population is becoming sexually active at a younger and younger age.

Work done by Nicholas Ford[2] is in agreement with that of many others in showing that teenagers are becoming sexually active at a very much younger age, and that over half of all the boys and girls surveyed were either sexually active on an ongoing basis, or have been sexually active by the age of sixteen. So they are very much at risk. If you then look at their sexual and contraceptive lifestyles, you can see where their risks of pregnancy, and their risks for infection, are coming from.

A third of these youngsters are using no method at all when they first start relationships. For those of us who work in family planning that will come as no surprise, because teenage sexual activity is notoriously unplanned and unprotected. Of those 40% who are using contraception, initially in relationships, barrier methods are often favoured, because the message about infections, because of the advent of HIV, is beginning to get across. Whereas, a much smaller percentage start off on the pill. When relationships last more than six months (and, of course, again, teenage relationships are notoriously short-lived) there is a change to this pattern – condoms become much less popular. This is certainly borne out in the clinic situations where one frequently sees young girls who are, say, six months into a relationship, and say 'Well, we're not entirely happy that the condom is safe enough to prevent pregnancy and we want to think about me changing on to the pill'. And this is evident by 42% using the pill.

But, of course, again, the pill does not protect against infections. In fact there is some evidence that the combined pill may cause eversion of the cervical columnar epithelium on to the ecto-cervix and this provides an ideal breeding ground for infections such as *Chlamydia*. And I am afraid the 'double Dutch' method, that is the method of using both the pill to stop a young girl getting pregnant and the condom to protect both partners from infections, has not yet caught on in Britain.

Another interesting point highlighted by Ford's study was that although intercourse was taking place within steady relationships there was also a significant level of sexual infidelity within such relationships – there was a fairly high level of partner change. So the scene is set for the consequences of not meeting sexual health needs; that is, pregnancy and infections. When you then see the age distribution of people attending the clinic where I work (at Withington in Manchester) it is not surprising to see that almost 40% of the people are under the age of 24 years[3]. And, in fact, 80% are under the age of 34. During 1991 and 1992 there were nearly 3500 cases of genital warts seen at our clinic and nearly 60% of those were in men and women under the age of 25. Now, you may say 'All right – well, warts are distressing, but they on the whole do not have any serious sequelae'. But, if you then look at *Chlamydia,* the story really becomes rather more alarming. Just over 2200 new cases in that same time period, and 60% of them were in young people under the age of 25. We all know the possible consequences of *Chlamydia* – endometritis, salpingitis, possible infertility and the personal anguish that it causes, and also the huge cost to the NHS. The same story is true of gonorrhoea, where, again, half of the cases are in young women. So we do have a problem. It is a problem that we must address.

It is a problem that is quite difficult to address and, certainly, there has been some resistance to sending people from family planning clinics and GP surgeries along to GUM departments. It is not the easiest thing to go along and talk about intimate things, but it is very important that we make sure people are referred to the right places. And, inevitably, women usually present with their vaginal discharge and genital warts to the family planning clinic rather than to the GUM clinic. Although things are changing and, although attendance at GUM clinics used to be very much in favour of men, that ratio is in fact now changing, and at our clinic we see more women than men.

So there is an overlap in clinical need. If women are coming along to family planning clinics it is essential that we have the facilities to screen for these infections, and if we do not have the facilities we know where to send those women. So, I would hope that most clinics and surgeries have not only the facilities for screening for vaginal infections, but also for endo-cervical infections like *Chlamydia* and gonorrhoea. And if you do not have those facilities, then it is important that you do send somebody somewhere else. How often have we seen the lady who says 'Oh, I had a discharge, I went along to see Dr X; he did a swab, it came back normal. I cannot have an infection'. But in many cases all that person has had is a high vaginal swab, so it is very important that comprehensive screening is done.

What happens next? It is very important that everybody has agreed referral protocols. I certainly think the message about *Chlamydia* has got across, but also women with genital warts must be referred to GUM clinics. It is a sexually transmitted infection. STDs are notoriously gregarious. They like going round in twos and threes, and so you must exclude other infections. Particularly, infections with more serious associations like trichomonas. In itself trichomonas is possibly not a terribly severe problem (although it can be a great nuisance), but it does have a high association with gonorrhoea; and it may well facilitate other infections being acquired.

Then we come to the personnel in GUM and family planning. It is essential that the personnel – nurses, doctors and counsellors in family planning – have knowledge of sexually transmitted infections. But it is equally important that the people who work in GUM have a high level of contraceptive awareness. It is an ideal time to do opportunistic family planning and opportunistic sexual health education. Again, when somebody has a problem they are at their most receptive to stopping that problem happening again. At the very minimum doctors working in GUM should possess their diploma in family planning and reproductive health care. It is important that both nurses and health advisers have knowledge of contraception. This is particularly so for the health advisers, because they are often the people who are giving the counselling and advice about contraception. So, continuing medical education is absolutely essential.

The way that we have achieved collaboration between the family planning services and the genitourinary services in South Manchester has really hinged on the shared personnel. When the GUM department was established in the mid-1980s, the nursing staff employed there were often the same nursing staff who worked in the family planning clinics. This tradition has continued and has had huge benefits both for the people who work in family planning and for the people who work in GUM clinics. And that has now been extended to the medical staff, whereby all the regular family planning doctors also have the opportunity to go and work in the GUM department for six months. The expertise that they gain is invaluable, and they bring that back to the family planning clinic. So the barriers between the two services have been broken down. Certainly, when we refer people either way, we are now confident that the service they are going to be given is a very effective and comprehensive one, but also delivered in a very non-judgemental way. So, that's one way we have of approaching the problem of meeting the sexual health needs of the women that we see.

Conclusion – Prof. Elstein

The message we would like to bring to you is about sex education. We are involved in looking at ways in which we can improve this in our region by linking up with the schools.

We also have established a young people's clinic and this has been very successful, and we have lots of young boys coming along. Interestingly enough, although the data are very small (because we do not swab every girl that comes in), among those girls of 16 or 17 years of age who have a discharge there is a very high prevalence rate of *Chlamydia*. In our clinics for young people we stress the importance of confidentiality. I urge you to look at the way in which you can provide this to the youngsters that are sexually active. And, of course, one has an opportunity to provide – what I call 'opportunistic health education'. We use the clinic waiting time for education in the ante-natal and gynaecological situations, and I think that we should do this much more widely.

Now, about the 'double Dutch' method – the pill and the condom. The Dutch seem to have got the message across. They have mainly a permissive and accepting attitude about sexuality. Their unplanned pregnancy rate among the young (under 19) is 4 per 1000, and 5 overall. Our figure for England and Wales is 21 for 16–19 year olds and 14 in women overall. If we are going to move healthcare-wise to the North American pattern, we have a worry. Their figures are appalling – 45 per 1000 for women aged 15–19 years and 28 overall. It is not advisable, therefore, to move across

11

the Atlantic in our attitudes and approach to this sort of problem.

So, what is the approach? This is the way we see it – a holistic one. Looking at the whole woman, and the whole family, looking at the service provision across the board and an integrated service. We believe that departments of obstetrics and gynaecology have a major role to play. We believe that GUM should be more related to the discipline of obstetric and gynaecology departments and should be part of their responsibility.

What is the way forward? Well, we think that the nursing and support staff should be trained in both areas and that the GP should be more involved. We should have community services, but there should also be a move towards the GP. We need to bring these skills to the GPs. We need to look at Well Women, but we must not forget the man as well.

References

1. Cates, W. (1984). Sexually transmitted diseases and family planning. Strange or natural bedfellows. *Journal of Reproductive Medicine,* **29**(5), 317–22.
2. Ford, N. (1993). Family planning and society: the sexual and contraceptive lifestyles of young people, Part 1. *British Journal of Family Planning,* **18**(3), 119–22.
3. *Annual Report* 1991/1992, Withington Hospital, Department of Genitourinary Medicine.

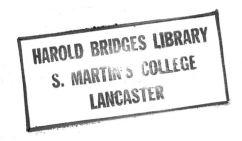
HAROLD BRIDGES LIBRARY
S. MARTIN'S COLLEGE
LANCASTER

2 Preliminary results from a short patient survey of sexual health promotion in genitourinary medicine clinics

Dr Jayshree Pillaye

This contribution presents the preliminary results from a short patient survey of sexual health promotion in GUM clinics. I would like to acknowledge the help and support given by the many health professionals working in GUM clinics and to express my thanks to those patients who participated in this survey.

The aim of the survey was to gauge patients' perception of their clinic visit, and whether they had information and services for wider sexual health promotion.

The method

Four GUM clinics were selected and two to three days were allocated for research in each one. The results are of those clinic attenders who agreed to participate in the survey on those days. The clinics were selected to give an adequate quota of patients from the minority ethnic communities, a varied prevalence of HIV, and also to have geographical variation so that they were not all in London.

A structured questionnaire was designed and patients were required to give a 'Yes' or 'No' response – with provision for making comments. Questions covered patients' views on posters, leaflets, discussion of safer sex – including the use of drugs and

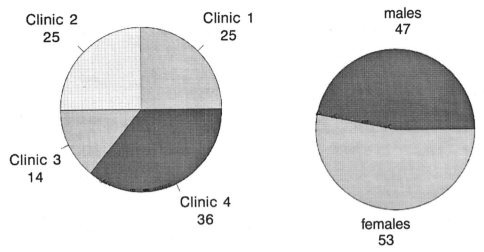

Fig 2.1: Percentage of respondents (N=449)

Fig 2.2: Gender of respondents (%)

alcohol, contraception, cervical smears, perception of visit and attitude to stigma and confidentiality.

The results

The total number of respondents was 449: 25% each from clinics 1 and 2, 14% from clinic 3 and 36% from clinic 4 (Fig. 2.1). Fifty-three per cent of the sample were females and 47% males (Fig. 2.2). When we look at the age breakdown it confirms both international and local findings, that most are under the age of 29 and about 8% are younger than 19 years. When we break these figures up further into age and gender, there are more females than males younger than 24 (Fig. 2.3).

Respondents were asked about their ethnicity and about 60% identified themselves

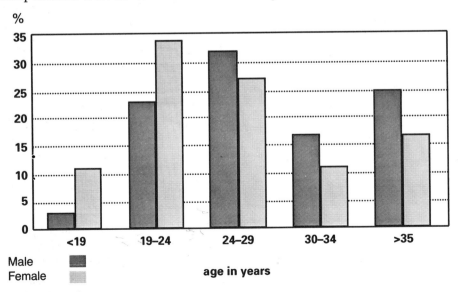

Fig 2.3: Age/gender

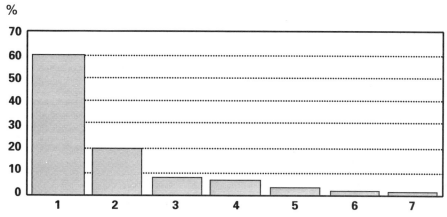

1=White British. 2=Afro-caribbean. 3=White others. 4=Black African.
5=Indian. 6=Pakistan and Bangladesh. 7=Chinese

Fig 2.4: Percentage distribution by ethnicity

as white British, about 8% white non-British, about 20% Afro-Caribbeans, about 6% Black Africans, about 2.5% Indians, 1% Chinese, and about 1.5% Pakistani and Bangladeshi (Fig. 2.4). I want to remind you that we did choose clinics to give an over-representation from the Black and minority ethnic communities, but further analysis is needed to see whether more people from the Afro-Caribbean and Black African communities attend STD clinics, and whether this is related to need or because they do not go to family planning clinics or to their GP.

About two-thirds of patients were either self-referral, or were referred by sources other than the GP. For about one-third it was their first visit.

Respondents were asked whether they were given any leaflets. About 30% said they had been, with about 29% responding that they had also received some explanation about them, mainly from the doctor or nurse. Just less than half (48%) said that they would have liked to have had some written information to take away with them. One patient, remarked,

> 'I do suggest that there should be leaflets to read in the waiting room. It seems that only the dregs of leaflets that no one wants are left lying about.'

Patients were then asked about condoms and whether they were offered any. About 49% were offered condoms to take away with them. About 21% received information on how to use them, with 9% saying that they received information on the use of spermicidal cream or pessaries (Fig. 2.5). About 45% would have preferred more condoms. Some would have also liked more information on condoms.

> 'I wanted to know about condoms, but they told me it was not necessary because I was getting the injection.'

We then asked about situational factors and whether this was discussed in regard to unsafe sex. About 20% reported that drugs as a factor leading to unsafe sex were discussed, while about 14% said that alcohol was discussed, and about 13% reported that both alcohol and drugs were discussed. Only about 15% were advised about hepatitis B vaccine (Fig. 2.6).

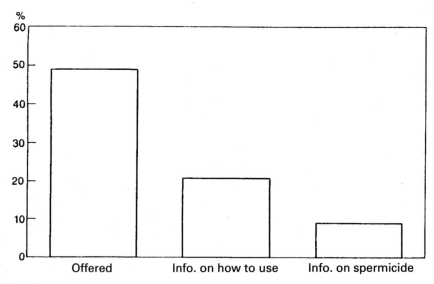

Fig 2.5: Condoms

Respondents were asked whether contraception was discussed – 35% of all the respondents answered affirmatively and the majority of these were female. Just fewer than half felt it was relevant for them to get this advice at a GUM clinic, and 62% felt that it would be more convenient for them to get this advice at a GUM clinic than a family planning clinic – again more females found this either relevant or convenient. When asked where they would go for follow-up contraception, about 55% said they would go to their GP and 67% of these were female. About 42% said they would go to

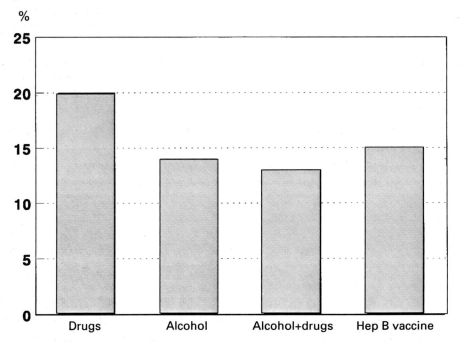

Fig 2.6: Percentage reporting discussion on various situational factors

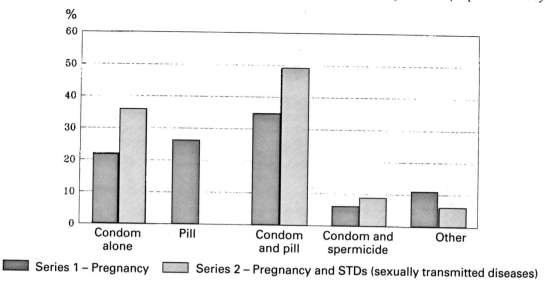

Fig 2.7: Methods used to prevent pregnancy and STDs

the family planning clinic and, again, more of these were female.

Respondents were also asked whether they would feel embarrassed to tell their GP or family planning clinic that they attended a GUM clinic. About 23% said they would be embarrassed to tell the GP and about 18% said they would be embarrassed to tell the family planning clinic.

When we come to the question of what patients would use either to prevent pregnancy or to prevent pregnancy and STDs, about 22% said they would use condoms alone to prevent pregnancies; 26% the pill alone; 35% the condom and the pill; 6% condom and spermicide; and 11% other methods – e.g. the coil and depo-provera injection and the rhythm method (Fig. 2.7).

When asked how they would avoid both STDs and pregnancy, 49% responded that they would use the condom and the pill; 36% would use the condom alone; 9% condoms and spermicide; and 6% other methods. So this sample of respondents did know about the double Dutch method and were actually using it.

Patients were asked about whether they knew about emergency contraception. About 76% of women knew, but about 54% of men responded that they had not heard about it. When asked where they could obtain it, 44% were aware that they could obtain it from the GP, 41% from the family planning clinic and only about 15% from the GUM clinic, and I would like to remind you that this is a GUM population (GUM clinic attenders) – this is worrying (Fig. 2.8).

About 70% of women reported that cervical smears were discussed with them, and about 5% had never had a smear. About half of the women said they would have liked more information about cervical smears. Women were then asked where they had had their smears done. About 14% had had their smears taken at the GUM clinic, about 57% at the GP surgery and about 7% at the family planning clinic. About 20% had had a smear at more than one of these clinics and only 2% had had it done by a gynaecologist or at an ante-natal clinic. When asked where would they prefer to have the smears taken 42% said at the GUM clinic, 39% at the GP surgery, 12% at the family

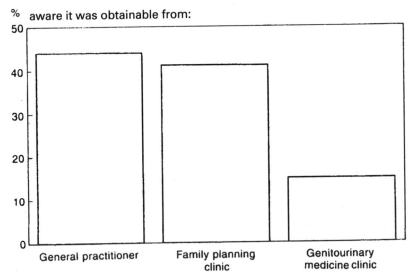

Fig 2.8: Knowledge of emergency contraception

planning clinic and 7% said they did not mind having it taken at any one of these clinics (Fig. 2.9).

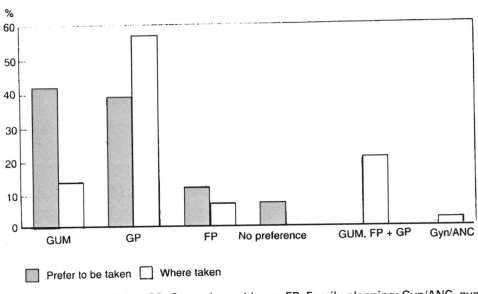

GUM= Genitourinary medicine; GP=General practitioner: FP=Family planning; Gyn/ANC=gynae-cology/ante-natal clinic

Fig 2.9: Cervical smears

We then asked about HIV infection and whether this had been discussed with them; 46% said no one had discussed HIV infection:

'*No information was given to me to take away; I would have liked some.*'

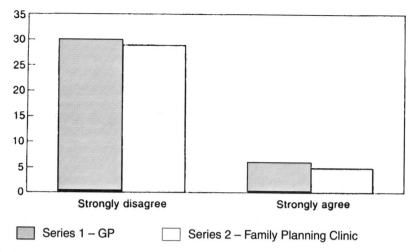

Fig 2.10: Patients asked if genitourinary medicine clinic should inform their doctor/family planning clinic about visit

'Nobody talked to me about HIV or AIDS.'

But, for a few, HIV and AIDS appeared to still instil a great anxiety:

'AIDS and HIV just freaks me out.'
'One big fear – I would rather not know; I will not have a test.'

Respondents were also asked whether they would be offended by clinic staff talking to them about HIV and AIDS, and about 5% said they would.

We then set out a series of statements, and patients were required to state how strongly they agreed or disagreed with each of them. We asked whether the GUM clinic should inform their doctor or the family planning clinic about their visit. About 30% strongly disagreed and 6% strongly agreed that the GUM clinic should inform their GP, and about 29% strongly disagreed and 5% strongly agreed that the GUM clinic should inform their family planning clinic about their visit (Fig. 2.10).

Patients were asked whether or not people should feel ashamed to attend a GUM clinic. About 49% strongly agreed that people should not feel ashamed to attend a GUM clinic and only about 1% strongly disagreed (Fig. 2.11).

About 54% strongly agreed that they should get all their sexual health promotion, tests and treatment at the GUM clinic. No one strongly disagreed.

About 15% strongly agreed – and the same proportion strongly disagreed – that the name GUM Clinic should be changed to sexual health clinic:

'People should not feel ashamed, but they do. The general image to most people is a place where people come to get rid of the clap; can anything be done to improve this?'

And there were many comments about doing something to remove the stigma that is associated with visiting a GUM clinic. For some:

'It's irrelevant to me what it's called; it used to be STD.'
'It makes no odds what it is called; it is the social inhibition that's the problem.'

19

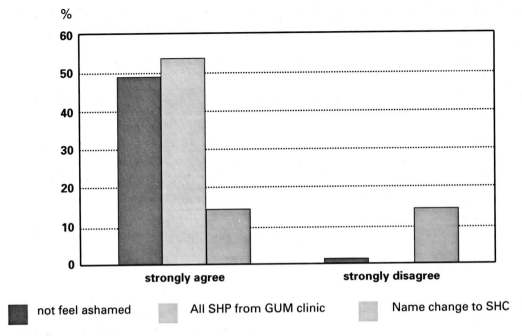

SHP=Sexual health promotion; SHC=Sexual health clinic

Fig 2.11: Stigma of visiting a GUM clinic

So, in summary, the patients who were interviewed wished to receive sexual health promotion at the GUM clinic visit. However, there still appeared to be some stigma attached to attending a GUM clinic, and clinic attenders did not wish others (including their GP) to know about their visit. However, although acknowledging the stigma, they did not feel it should be a barrier once they actually attended the GUM clinic. Just under 50% of the patients received no information on HIV and AIDS. Reasons for this may include, that: many of the patients did not see a health adviser, when it was presumed that they had; patients came for specific treatments – for example, treatment of warts or for a colposcopy; health professionals did not think that it was necessary; or there may be lack of time both from the patient's and from the health professional's side.

Men who identified themselves as gay felt that they were receiving inadequate information on safer sex. A few also felt that some doctors were not so comfortable with them. Some of the comments made:

'I would like to know more about the infections gay men can get, but all the leaflets are for heterosexual sex.'
'Not enough information; I had to ask specific questions about safer sex.'
'I definitely would like more information on gay safer sex.'

The few Asian women seen either used a coil or were on depo-provera, and they received no information on HIV infection or condom use. Many women commented that they wanted more information on cervical cancer and colposcopy.

'I would like more information on cancer of the cervix and colposcopy. I had a

colposcopy two times before – both were positive. I became pregnant and could not have treatment because I was pregnant. No one told me that the pregnancy would delay treatment.'

'Herpes – cervical cancer – tests. I did not know anything about tests or why they were taken; they just took them.'

'What can be found out with a smear? Example – AIDS? Or do you have to have an additional test?'

And more generally, patients wanted to know what would happen to them when they attended a GUM clinic. Who will they see? In what order? And how long will their visit probably last? But, many patients did comment that they were happy with the service:

'No need for improvement.'

'Excellent service.'

'This is the first time I've attended, but I was quite satisifed.'

Conclusion

The aim of the survey was to gauge patients' perceptions of their clinic visit. Many did not know what to expect on their first visit, and some of them had some difficulty in distinguishing between the health professionals. Some were confused about why they were seeing the health adviser and why they had to see both a nurse and a health adviser. They also wanted more information about the reasons for tests being done. Many, especially women, wanted to know how long were they likely to spend at the clinic?

This survey has highlighted the need for more patient information about HIV infection, cervical smears and colposcopy. Gay men wanted more information on safer sex. The majority of patients wanted to receive sexual health education and information, tests and treatment at the GUM clinic. While acknowledging there was some stigma attached to visiting a GUM clinic, there was a plea to de-stigmatise it.

3

A sexual health service under one roof

Peter Greenhouse

It is a matter of some concern that no concise, widely understood and accepted definition of sexual health yet exists, some two years after the launch of *The Health of the Nation,* and three years after the term gained widespread currency with the conference report *Promoting Sexual Health*[1]. In this contribution, I aim to offer a definition of sexual health, consider the reasons why people have sex, and thereby describe the services required to meet their needs. I will examine the unequal burden of health problems faced by women and men, review the history of service development and highlight the exceptional damage to (mostly women's) health caused by artificial barriers in service provision. Finally, I shall discuss logistics and operational problems in running a sexual health service, and identify some of the absolute obstacles to progress.

Definition

> *Sexual health is the enjoyment of sexual activity of one's choice, without causing or suffering physical or mental harm*[2].

This statement can be interpreted as uniting all the positive aspects of sex as a life-enhancing source of self-fulfilment and pleasure given by mutual consent, be it heterosexual, gay or lesbian sex. It includes, of course, the safest form of sexual expression – masturbation – and also the option of no activity – abstinence – as a positively healthy choice.

It implies responsibility, both for self and others, in adopting behaviour which will reduce risk of damage, such as unwanted pregnancy, infection, genital cancer, etc. It emphasises the need to consider mental health as an integral part of sexual health, and can highlight such obvious combinations of physical and psychological harm, such as sexual assault, abortion, dyspareunia and infertility. I commend the definition to you and welcome constructive criticism.

✳ *Motivation*

Why do people bother to have sex? The vast majority of adolescents and young adults are sexually active (whether by choice or not) and have no immediate desire to conceive, whilst wishing to preserve their future potential fertility. The fortunate ones choose to have sex for recreation not procreation; for the unfortunates, it is a matter of coercion or survival. Most will spend some considerable time discovering exactly what they want to do, and with whom they wish to do it.

Recreation represents choice; coercion or survival, no choice. Pleasure instead of pain. Fun not fear. Freedom or slavery. Enjoyment versus employment. Natural desires rather than market forces.

Current problems

Although most people spend very little time during their lives having sex for procreation, conventional gynaecology devotes the bulk of its resource to serving this relatively infrequent activity, largely ignoring the reality of recreational, commercial or traumatic sex in its patient population. This imbalance must be redressed when designing sexual health care services which, locally, not only take the lead in preventive education, promoting the positive aspects of behavioural choice in relationships for both women and men, but provide contraception, barrier protection and STD care, and deal with the widest range of serious health problems of sexual activity. Looking at the cumulative prevalence of principal sexual health problems by age 40 in the UK (Fig. 3.1), we can see that harm (accidental or intentional) occurs more frequently and seriously to women through their contact with men than vice versa. Women bear the burden of man's excess – both literally and metaphorically. Any infection is more likely to be transmitted from man to women, due to anatomical vulnerability.

At least one-third of women will have had a termination of pregnancy. This figure hides an unknown number of women who continued their unwanted pregnancies, and, of course, the unseen number of men who caused them. Studies from the USA and Sweden calculate that 30–50% of women now aged 40 will have had one episode of salpingitis, with the resultant possibility of infertility, principally because of the covert sexually transmitted agent *Chlamydia*.

Although I shall concentrate on these two issues, one must not ignore the other three major problems – psychosexual trauma, cervical premalignancy and HIV. There is no known research in the world which shows a prevalence of sexual abuse in any

1. Terminated pregnancy	40
2. Salpingitis	30
3. Psycho-sexual trauma	>10
4. Cervical (pre)malignancy	5
5. HIV	<0.5
(approx. cumulative prevalence by age of 40)	

Fig 3.1: Principal sexual health problems (%)

female population studied of less than 10%. Some 5% of women will have had abnormal cytology, the figure rising to 10% in STD clinics. Inadequate care of women with HIV has thrown the spotlight on the traditional areas of clinical and social neglect which are the subject of this contribution.

Service needs

Let us consider the possible medical service needs (Fig. 3.2) of a young, sexually active woman who has no wish to conceive – namely contraception, abortion or infection care. In the picture 'Black Magic' (1935) by René Magritte (see pl. 1), medical attention is concentrated below the umbilicus, while the real damage (psychological) is going on above the neck, with little or no notice taken. Sexual health services must specifically address *both* medical and psychological needs in an empathetic, holistic fashion.

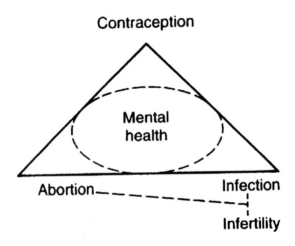

Fig 3.2: Sexual health care needs

A considerate, non-judgemental philosophy is fundamental to creating a secure, acceptable and supportive environment for each woman (or man) at a time when they feel most vulnerable. If we concentrate provision from a team of specialised and sympathetic staff, this ensures consistent clinical management, and reduces overheads. Therefore, the most efficient arrangement for both cost and convenience is to place all the services, including contraception and abortion, STD and HIV, cytology, colposcopy and vulvoscopy, sexual assault care and psychosexual dysfunction, counselling and community sexual health promotion, under one roof.

Improving the sexual health of the nation, demands a substantial effort directed at bettering young women's health, which is the principal target of our own locally expanded service. Although we can see in Magritte's picture 'The Ready-made Bouquet' (1936) (see pl. 2) that women's problems are more obvious, most derive from the man behind – little real progress will be made if we ignore him. Although this is a far more difficult and specialised task, one could improve women's lot substantially by concentrating education and care entirely on heterosexual men. If successful, are we to believe

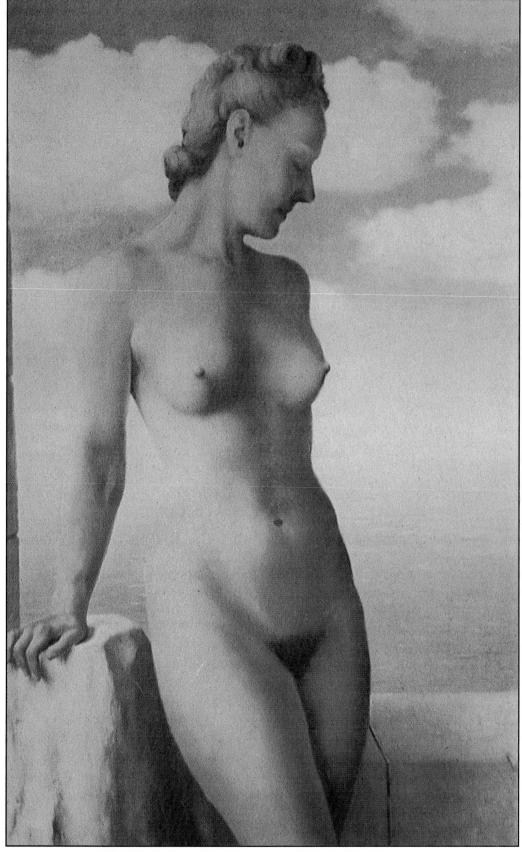

Plate 1   *Leitmotif* for holistic sexual health care (physical and mental).
La Magie Noir (Black Magic).1935. René Magritte.
©ADAGP, Paris and DACS, London 1994.

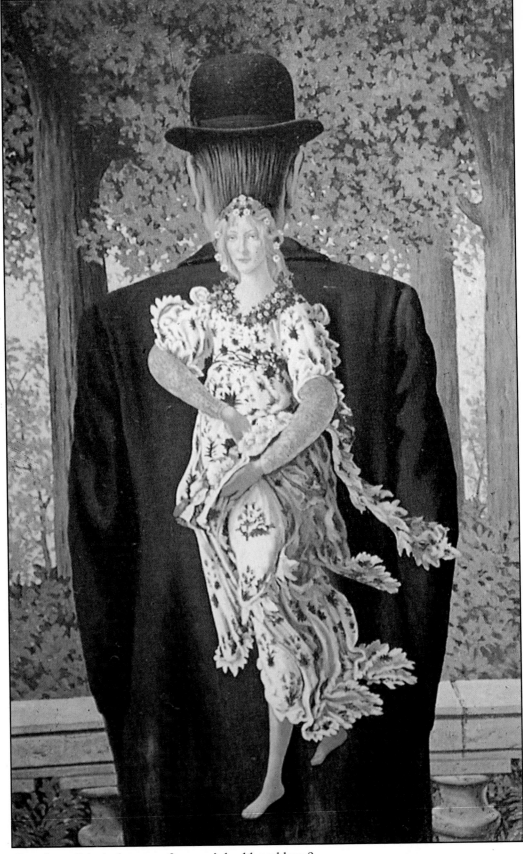

Plate 2   Principal source of women's health problems?
Le Bouquet Tout-Fait (The Ready-made Bouquet).1956. René Magritte.
©ADAGP, Paris and DACS, London 1994.

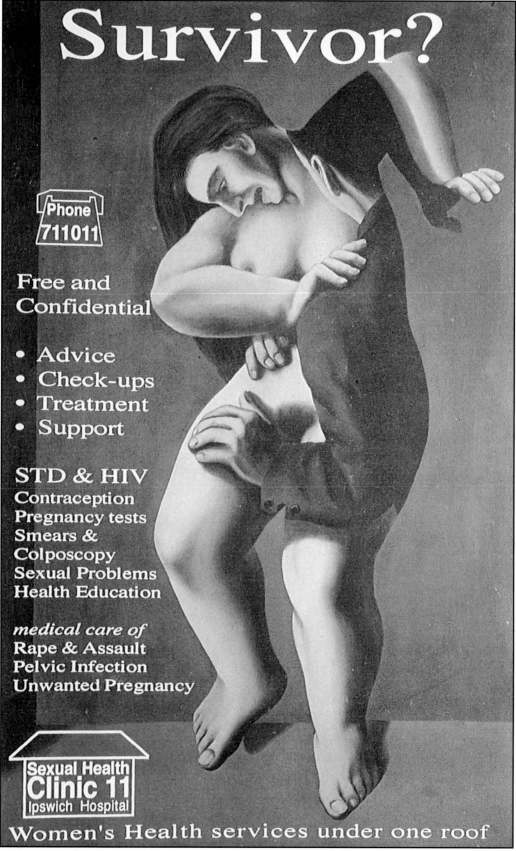

Plate 3   Supportive services for survivors.
Poster based on *Les Jours Gigantesques (Titanic Days)*.1928. René Magritte.
©ADAGP, Paris and DACS, London 1994.

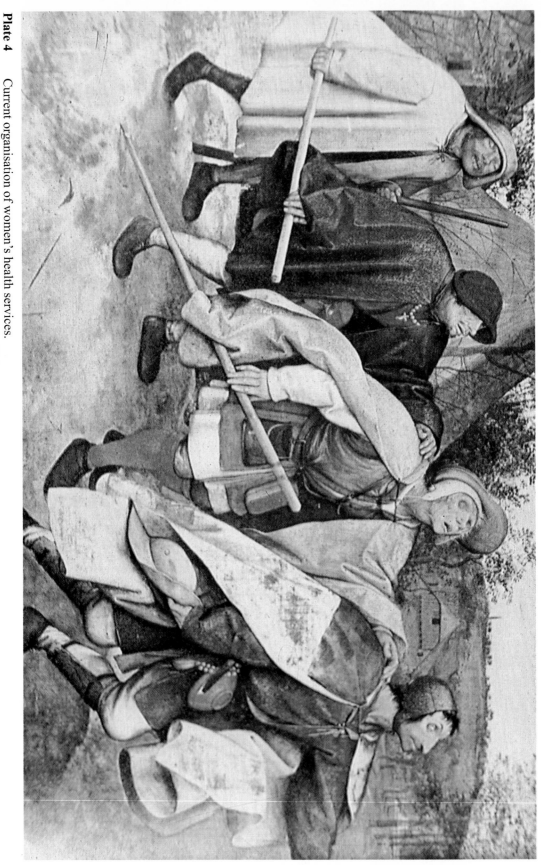

Plate 4 Current organisation of women's health services. *The Parable of the Blind*.1568. Pieter Bruegel the Elder. Musée du Louvre, Paris.

that we could so reduce the prevalence of infection in men, and improve their under-standing and attitude toward women that they may no longer constitute a threat to women's health? – I fear not.

Mind the gap

Despite recent developments, most genitourinary physicians have little or no training in women's health care, and the vast majority of gynaecologists are ignorant of STDs. Young women fall into huge gaps of service provision, artificial constraint and igno-rance between gynaecology, family planning, general practice and genitourinary medi-cine. They face an endless traipse from one doctor to another having different aspects of the same problem sorted out in an inconsistent and sometimes inconsiderate fashion. This is an unspeakable waste of time, energy, emotion and medical resource – the very disparate nature of current services not only prevents appropriately trained doctors from functioning effectively, but also causes frustration and degradation of women, leading to misery, morbidity and mismanagement, particularly in the inadequate care of unwanted pregnancy and lack of partner treatment for women with salpingitis.

Women have a justifiable right not to be exposed to clinicians who openly express patronising, disdainful or moralistic views on their sexual behaviour. Such rights would seem rarely to be respected outside GUM and contraception services – ask almost *any* woman who has sought termination of pregnancy.

A changing specialty

The specialty which others currently call GUM was created in 1917 by the second most sensible piece of public health legislation ever enacted (second only to the Abortion Act). It provided the UK with free and entirely confidential clinics in every major town, for the control, diagnosis and treatment of STD, which remains unique in the world. The pattern of disease and attendance at the clinics has changed dramatically over the last 50 years, reflecting demographic change, war, travel, contraceptive practice and sexual mores.

There was a wartime peak of gonorrhoea (Fig. 3.3) in 1945–6. War is the greatest aphrodisiac – 'if you're going to die tomorrow . . . what are you doing tonight?' This is

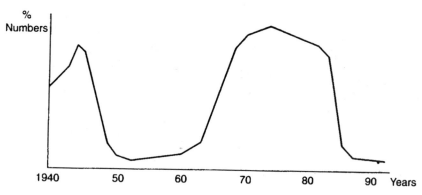

Fig 3.3: Trends in UK clinic reports of gonorrhoea

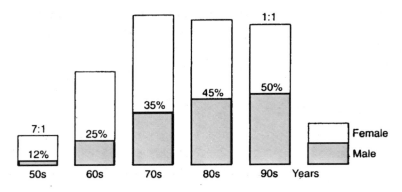

Fig 3.4: Proportion of women seen in clinics compared to men

followed by a rapid drop with the arrival of penicillin and post-war reactionary morality, with the 1950s (the 'Back-to-Basics' period) being a somewhat frustrating time for young people. The tremendous rise in STDs in the 1960s is well recognised, with the post-war baby boom reaching adolescence, a gradual change in sexual behaviour and slow uptake of fertility control, but the 1970s and early 1980s were more significant. Having the highest ever rates of STD and contraceptive pill use, my generation of teenagers suffered unsympathetic, inadequate care – in general practice and gynaecology – from those doctors who had themselves been teenagers in the restricted years of the 1950s. Much psychological damage was caused, principally to young women, by older, moralistic male doctors.

The specialty had been almost exclusively concerned with male patients, with male to female ratios around 7:1 in the early 1950s (Fig. 3.4). This changed to 4:1 in 1960, 2:1 in 1970, reaching parity in some clinics by the mid-1980s. Yet training in gynaecology was not 'required' for junior doctors until 1986.

Reviewing actual workload in 1992–3 at Ipswich (Fig. 3.5), although there were 50:50 new women to men, two-thirds of follow-ups were for women, with 70% of the drug bill (excluding HIV care) on women. Women had three-quarters of all tests,

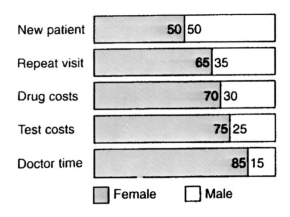

Fig 3.5: Clinic workload by sex of patient

because of the number of sites to be sampled. Thus, some *85% of doctors' clinical time is now devoted to care of women* whereas this same proportion of effort was expended on men some 40 years ago. This pattern is typical of other medium-size provincial services, but varies with the interest and reputation of each clinic.

Similar clientele, younger risk

Consider the age distribution of female sexual health/GUM clinic attenders (Fig. 3.6). Ninety per cent of all infections are acquired before age 25 – so, if you have not had a 'dose' by the time you are 30, you have not been trying hard enough! Or you have

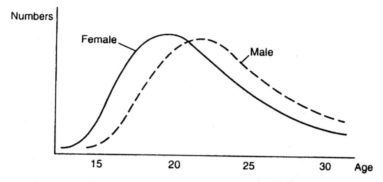

Fig 3.6: Age and sex profile of sexually transmitted disease clinic attenders

never had any symptoms, and you have never been checked for infection. This has a most important bearing on 'well woman' services, where, particularly in the 15–24 age group, a well woman is one who has had a smear, but does not realise that she has not been tested for a treatable infection which could easily be present and might make her infertile, for example *Chlamydia*.

If we wish to turn STD incidence into true prevalence, the denominator *should* consist of only those individuals at risk – i.e. some 30% of 15-year-olds, and 95%+ of women aged 20, giving a more frightening but accurate picture (Fig. 3.7). Adolescents are the group most vulnerable to sexual health problems: false impressions of immor-

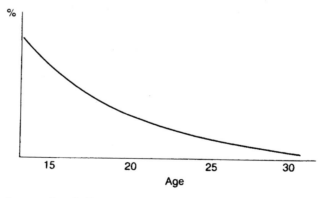

Fig 3.7: Sexually transmitted disease prevalence adjusted for sexual activity

27

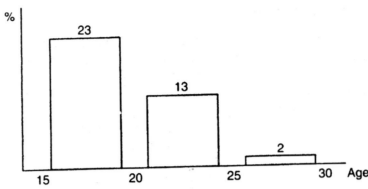

Fig 3.8: *Chlamydia* prevalence at abortion

tality, unbounded energy, desire for new experience and peer and media pressure, all create an enthusiastic drive for risk taking around sex and drugs. Those who are sexually active aged under 20 have the *highest rates of unwanted pregnancy and STD acquisition* (including HIV), of any group in the population.

The other contributors have alluded to the fact that women attending either contraception, abortion or infection clinics have, as expected, similar backgrounds of sexual activity and experience[3], and virtually identical rates of STD. Some studies show higher prevalence of STD in younger women requesting abortion, which is predictable, as the youngest girls, if sexually active, have the highest risk of infection (Fig. 3.8). In 1986[4], almost one-quarter of women under the age of 20 having abortions, were infected with *Chlamydia*. At this time, nationally, less than one per cent of women were routinely screened pre-operatively for infection. The resulting magnitude of iatrogenic salpingitis and consequent infertility may never be fully appreciated.

There is a clear need for full sexual health care to be built into abortion services. Women need time to discuss fears and weigh decisions, arrange future contraception, be screened pre-operatively for infection, and have continuity of follow-up. This may best be achieved by taking abortion services out of the hands of routine gynaecology altogether or providing all care, apart the actual operation, from a sexual health/GUM or contraception service.

Lost opportunities

I once had the misfortune to work in a GUM clinic which displayed an old Durex poster where you could see that the words 'contraception and' had been blanked out from the caption 'Ask here for advice on *[contraception and]* protection from sexually transmitted diseases'. That GUM clinics should have taken active steps to prevent contraceptive care is as indefensible as the lost opportunity of some one million women being seen annually in family planning clinics without widespread access to *Chlamydia* screening and treatment.

In a recent audit over a three-month period at Charing Cross Hospital[3], four per cent of all women who had recently attended the GUM clinic became pregnant, two-thirds being unplanned. This and the above provide a powerful argument for complete integration of contraception and GUM facilities at the same sites, under the banner of Sexual Health.

What's in a name?

'Family planning' is for people who are planning not to have families – enough said.

Our sexual health clinic offers a service for people who have sex and want to stay healthy. This is an easily understandable name which reflects an important, sex positive, health seeking message. The major shift in emphasis is away from the clinic you only use when there is something wrong, to being the place you go regularly to make sure you are healthy. As most major STDs are asymptomatic (often until it is too late), anything which promotes preventive health care or early clinical presentation is to be encouraged.

On my appointment (1991), the Ipswich STD clinic immediately dispensed with the name genitourinary medicine, which has always been totally meaningless or misleading to the public, and has little or no currency with health promoters or personal and social education (PSE) teachers (let alone among many of our medical colleagues). Its negative imagery, redolent of genitalia and urine, compounded any perceived stigma, increased confusion, and could only hinder the accessibility or acceptability of the service. It would be unfortunate if this term were to survive the decade.

So what's new?

In addition to the existing basic STD and HIV services, we immediately set up full colposcopy and vulvoscopy diagnosis and treatment, on-site pregnancy testing, formal medical work-up and counselling prior to termination referral, and contraception provision. This was only possible because of adequate nursing and medical staffing levels and appropriate previous training. Our work complements and supports existing gynaecology services, particularly with a unified colposcopy management protocol, and immediate out-patient access for pelvic pain assessment, exclusion of infection and partner screening for cases of suspected salpingitis. We also had the exceptional good fortune to move into new accommodation and inherit unused colposcopy equipment.

We tried to create a more supportive environment by giving the nurses greater responsibility for individual patients, and harnessing their natural communication skills and empathy. All staff were trained at the National AIDS Counselling Training Unit (NACTU), some took psychosexual courses or health education degrees, and seem to have been motivated and empowered by the metamorphosis from former chaperons or technicians into practitioners and counsellors. From the patients, there followed an increasing number of first revelations of previous sexual assault, for which we offer a triage service in close collaboration with psychologists working with sexual trauma and dysfunction. (For poster advertising services to survivors of sexual assault, see pl. 3.)

The scope of our sexual health facilities can be contrasted with another type of GUM clinic – anonymous – which considers its women's health remit to be 'very good at sorting out vaginal discharge and non-specific urethritis (NSU) contacts, but not much else'.

Health promotion from a sexual health clinic

Although the area of sexual health promotion which occurs *within* GUM clinics has been considered in other contributions, we assume, like others, that careful communication with patients has always been an essential part of our work. Our clinic is the principal local source both of care and authoritative information on sexual health; and our public health role is the control of STD in the community, so we have taken a lead in sexual health education. We run an extensive lecturing and seminar programme to staff, volunteers, schools and other public groups, with some 100 teaching activities in the last academic year. An increasing number of secondary schools have requested our input both to planning course content and by direct teaching of 14- to 18-year-olds. This provides the triple benefit of supporting teaching staff, assisting in the broader context of youth health promotion, and advertising clinical services to, and raising awareness among, the current and future population at risk. A recent Department for Education schools inspectorate report described the input as being 'of exceptionally high quality'.

An important national and local initiative has been the attempt to integrate pure, isolated HIV education, fully into sexual health promotion. Although in other areas of health promotion you might be able to persuade people to give up the drink before and the cigarette after, the desirability and universality of what occurs in between, demands that sexual health education be delivered by staff who have specialised personal skills of communication, open-mindedness, lack of moralising and practical experience of the subject, without which credibility is easily undermined. It is no good if you have only learned it from a book.

We would suggest, to achieve maximum cost benefit, service cohesion (and credibility), that sexual health education be separated from less controversial areas of health promotion, and is best delivered by an educator working within a clinical background, as part of the care delivery team. This ensures that a clear, accurate, comprehensible and empowering message is communicated, which is consistent with the advice which will be given during clinical care.

Certainly, putting community sexual health promotion and sexual health clinical provision together would be a tremendous cost saving in terms of non-duplication of resource materials. It would be mutually beneficial for care-givers and educators, and you would end up with a better quality product. I think that is what people want.

Theory

We need to bridge the gap between GUM, contraception and gynaecology, creating a service which fully addresses the needs of sexually active women and their partners. This requires a breakdown of rigid specialty divisions, giving improved clinical continuity and convenience for patients, and preventing iatrogenesis due to ignorance. Most developments have to be low- or no-cost, and can be achieved by collaboration in training of existing staff, most efficiently by in-house teaching in each other's disciplines, and by untying the hands of those already trained between the three areas. Althoughy the cost of (say) contraception in GUM clinics, or vice versa, may appear substantial to a large inner-city clinic, an overall cost benefit to the district should accrue by preventing multiple service attendances by the same woman. There should also be a cost opportunity of treating or preventing closely-associated problems, by accessing a larger proportion of the at-risk population at several different sites.

Reality

In attempting to provide 'everything' under one roof, local circumstances and individual initiative will obviously dictate the limits of what is logistically or politically possible. This must be balanced with the need to provide access widely across the community, hence the overriding need for a consistent clinical management philosophy of sexual health care between complementary primary and secondary services.

So what can we do? It would be simple to stick the whole lot under one roof in one department, but this would dramatically reduce accessibility. Perhaps in the inner city you could do it, but in a rural area such as mine you have to enlist the help of the family planning clinics, which could combine the best of both services. They will still continue to give the good contraceptive and cytology care they gave before, but it will be just that bit more effective. The minimum requirement is to get proper STD and HIV advice into these clinics, achieved by mutual staff training, in addition to *Chlamydia* screening, and limited antibiotic dispensing.

We also enlist our general practitioners (GPs) because, in a large rural area, where patients can be 40 miles away, there are some excellent GPs in the community who have empathy for young people and a high standard of STD knowledge. They are effectively running their own community STD services as satellites from the main clinic. I think this should be encouraged more widely.

Before going any further, I think it is self-evident that if you are a women, from the point of view of a professional woman care-giver, a women recipient, or a potential recipient of care you should be interested in advocating this type of service (be it in the community or in hospital). After all, *your* fertility could be at risk. Unfortunately, men are not so seriously threatened by sexual health problems. It does not matter so much to them. Yet men are in control of most of the money and service delivery. So, whether you like it or not, we face a problem of medical and sexual politics.

Obstacles

It is a sad reflection of the status of women in society, that in the only area of women's health controlled by women, namely 'family planning', they had been so completely disempowered that they were unable to prescribe anything other than contraception. Even now, many do not demand their rights to wider clinical freedom, despite the undoubted benefits which would accrue to their patients.

I have alluded to the historical barriers to effective sexual health care. These include the curiously British traditional attitude to sex, of simultaneous prurience and prudishness, double-standard morality and misogyny, born of an erstwhile sex and generation gap between doctors and patients, which, mercifully has disappeared in all but the highest echelons of power.

Perhaps an important obstacle has been the Royal College of Obstetricians and Gynaecologists' 12-year delay in recognition of the specialty of reproductive health/medical gynaecology. It remains unclear as to how much interest the new faculty will take in the control of STD in gynaecology, or, indeed in non-reproductive sex in general.

A significant minority of GPs also play their part. Some do not seem to understand patients' fundamental rights to alternative primary sources of care for sexual issues, in particular the legal guarantee of confidentiality in GUM clinics, without which patients would not disclose sensitive details. Many clinics actively and successfully invite women to consent to important information (on cytology or threats to fertility) being passed to the GP in the interests of continuity of care. Consent here depends primarily on the woman's trust in her GP's attitude. This effort has recently been damaged by the insurance industry's stance on HIV risk assessment [this has now changed, i.e. the insurance agencies have reviewed their policy), although locally we have circumvented the problem with those GPs who use a standard disclaimer for 'lifestyle' questions.

Other GPs may feel threatened by competition, and some are particularly vexed by antibiotic dispensing in contraception centres. This attitude is often associated with an inability to discuss or even consider sexual problems when dealing with patients (who therefore choose confidential, specialised sexual health services – Ed.], or the tremendously variable standard of STD teaching in medical schools, or perhaps commercial pressures. This might be mitigated by better access to and regulation of contraception and STD training for GPs and practice nurses.

So, while women may be crying out for better quality services, most resistance has come from men, perhaps even from those who control gynaecology and GUM, thereby controlling most of women's health care. Some will say that these new, integrated services might be expensive in the short term, without looking to the longer health gain. I have no idea of any hidden agendas or vested interests, but, certainly, the way services have hitherto been designed looks rather like the picture 'The Parable of the Blind' (1562) Pieter Bruegel the Elder (see pl. 4).

There may be light at the end of the tunnel. As more women with HIV present to gynaecologists, they are likely to force a change in service provision and training. A woman with HIV (or indeed any other vulnerable woman) should expect absolute confidentiality, absolute consideration and absolute consistency and expertise in her care. She may not wish to see a physician who knows little about gynaecology, nor a gynaecologist who knows little about infection. Gynaecological services will have to improve the level of care provided, increasing the training of staff in HIV and other aspects of women's sexual health, which, if applied widely, may reduce the current neglect of sexual problems across the entire population served. This might even help prevent some HIV.

Conclusions

In summary, I would like to see sexual health services under one roof in order to maximise resources and minimise the harm done to women. I have tried to do it locally in a very small way, and there are others around the country who are working towards a similar ideal. Women are entitled to civilised standards of sympathy, consideration and non-judgemental medical and nursing care whether they are having sex for recreation or reproduction, coercion or survival. As we have seen, the reality falls woefully short of this ideal. If, according to Philip Larkin 'sexual intercourse began in 1963' then the development of women's health services to respond to this challenge is already 30 years too late. Medicine has failed a generation of women.

The exceptional needs of women with HIV may at last force conventional gynaecological services to make better provision for all sexually active women. Logistics may be difficult, traditionally entrenched obstacles remain daunting. However, I put it to you that the arguments for holistic sexual health care, be they economic, personal convenience or public health, have always been strong and are now overwhelming. Perhaps the only way we will advance is if women's health is both decided and provided *by* women *for* women.

References

1. Hendriks, A. (1992). The political and legislative framework in which sexual health promotion takes place. In *Promoting Sexual Health,* (ed) Curtis, H. ch.21, p.156. British Medical Association Foundation for AIDS, London.
2. Greenhouse, P. (1994). Under one roof: Setting up sexual health services for women. *Maternal and Child Health,* **19,** 228–33.
3. Radcliffe, K. W. *et al.* (1993). A comparison of sexual behaviour and risk behaviour for HIV infection between women in three clinical settings. *Genitourinary Medicine* **69,** 441–5.
4. Fish, A. N. J. (1989). Chlamydial infection in women: clinical and epidemiological studies. MD Thesis. University of London.

4

A women's only session in a genitourinary medicine clinic

Dr Fiona Boag

This contribution presents details about the women-only session held within our GUM clinic, providing integrated health care including advice, counselling and information on sexually transmitted infections, HIV and family planning.

I was asked to start this clinic mainly by the receptionists who told me that people phoned up, either women or their male partners, wanting to come to the clinic and if we could not guarantee that the lady would be seen by female staff, the lady would not come. HIV-positive women also suggested they would prefer some of their services to be provided in a female environment. Doctors and nurses working within the clinic said

Table 4.1. Views of 50 HIV antibody-positive women attending our genitourinary medicine (GUM) and HIV out-patient clinics

	Numbers	
Discomfort felt attending GUM clinic	0	(0%)
Discomfort felt attending HIV clinic	10	(20%)
Preference for a female-only clinic	16	(32%)
Preference for a female-only HIV clinic	23	(46%)
Wanted a social worker, health adviser and dietitian to be available	43	(86%)
Requested crèche facilities	0	(0%)

that there was a need for a women's clinic. There were patients where the doctors found it hard to get to the root of their problems, who felt such a service would be beneficial. Doctors and nurses from our clinic – e.g. family planning doctors, GPs, and gynaecologists – also felt such a service would be valuable. Self-help groups also supported the idea.

We surveyed 50 HIV-positive women (Table 4.1) who were attending our services; they did not feel uncomfortable attending the mixed-sex GUM clinic, but we do not feel that is the best place for them to receive their health care, because it is a walk-in clinic with different doctors all the time. Twenty per cent felt discomfort attending the dedicated HIV clinic known as the Kobler Centre; mainly, we think because most of the patients were men. There was a preference for a women's clinic and a preference for the social workers, health advisers and dietitian to be available.

We then surveyed a small number of women who were attending a self-help group (Table 4.2) and many of them were not attending any clinic for health care. They had been diagnosed HIV-positive, and gone back maybe once or twice to the clinic but were no longer receiving care. Many of these women also had children. There was a strong request for a female-based clinic with integrated family planning, gynaecology and smears. They also wanted counsellors and support services/support group to be available.

Table 4.2. HIV clinic facilities preferred by 18 HIV antibody-positive women attending a self-help group

	Numbers	
Integrated family planning, gynaecology and cervical cytology	18	(100%)
Social worker available	18	(100%)
Crèche facilities	18	(100%)
A female doctor	15	(83%)
Counsellor available	14	(78%)
An integrated support group	13	(72%)
Female patients only	9	(50%)
All female staff	6	(33%)

We, therefore, set about providing such a service. As we did not have enough HIV-positive women to have a clinic just for them, we decided we would integrate STD screening, testing and ongoing care in a booked clinic. For logistical reasons, we hold this in the evening, because we obviously cannot shut during the day. Initially, the service was provided by volunteers – women volunteered their services to work one evening a week. Family planning came on board after the service had been running for about 18 months, by which time, we had convinced our purchasers that the service was worth paying for, so we were able to bring in a few more staff.

The substance misuse service was with us for about a year, but withdrew due to

Dr Fiona Boag

poor uptake of services, as did the paramedical support. The counsellor/health adviser is still needed all the time, but the dietitian, paediatric nurse, social worker and so forth are available if requested by the patients, but do not come every week. Psychosexual medicine is also provided in the same way.

Table 4.3. Reasons for attending a women-only clinic*

	Number	
Female doctor	69	(62.2%)
Female clinic staff	56	(50.4%)
Evening clinic	47	(47.3%)
Female patients only	39	(35.0%)
Child care easier†	21	(18.9%)

n: total number of women = 111.
* Groups are not mutually exclusive.
† All women with small children indicated that childcare was easier.

After the first six months, we looked at the reasons why the women said they were attending the clinic (Table 4.3). There were many reasons, but they did focus around the female staff and the female patients in the waiting room. They felt more comfortable sitting with women. The women with children found it easier to arrange for someone to look after their family during the evening. An evening clinic was also very popular – many of our women go out to work and have very busy schedules, and find it difficult to excuse themselves from work to go to a clinic for sexual health needs. We provide a mixed clinic in an evening on another day, so that we are providing equal services for men.

Table 4.4. Choice of alternative site in the absence of a women-only clinic

	Number	
Total women asked	73	(100%)
Well woman clinic	21	(28.8%)
Mixed-sex GUM clinic	32	(43.8%)
GP or FPC	10	(13.7%)
Don't know	7	(9.6%)
Nowhere	3	(4.0%)

GUM: genitourinary medicine; GP: general practitioner;
FPC: family planning clinic.

If we had not provided the women's clinic, less than half of the women said they would not have gone to a mixed-sex GUM clinic (Table 4.4). Some would not know

where to go or would not have gone anywhere, or they would have gone to GPs, family planning clinics, or well woman clinics. Maybe, they would have been satisfied atte-dending other services, but we found that when we compared the sexually transmitted infections found in the first 65 patients attending our clinic (Table 4.5) with women attending the GUM clinic (the John Hunter Clinic) we found that more of our patients had warts – although our numbers were small, we were finding more *Chlamydia* and more herpes than in the normal GUM clinic. Overall, the STD rate was similar. Since this time, we have now seen more *Trichomonas* than in the mixed sex clinic as well, and we have seen some scabies and syphilis.

Table 4.5. Sexually transmitted infections in women attending the women-only clinic (WOC) and John Hunter Clinic (JHC)

	Infections (WOC n=65)	Diagnosed (JHC n=1567*)	
Candidosis	27 (41.5%)	350 (22.3%)	p < 0.001
Genital warts	22 (33.9%)	252 (16.1%)	p < 0.001
Chlamydia	6 (9.2%)	63 (4.0%)	
Genital herpes	5 (7.7%)	73 (4.7%)	
Bacterial vaginosis	4 (6.2%)	144 (9.2%)	
Gonorrhoea	1 (1.5%)	21 (1.3%)	
Trichomonas	0 (0%)	23 (1.5%)	
Sabies or pediculosis	0 (0%)	8 (0.5%)	
Syphilis	0 (0%)	3 (0.2%)	

* KC60 diagnosis of new women attending the John Hunter Clinic in 1991.

Who are these women? Are they really just the women that would have come to the clinic anyway? I do not think so. We have had twice the number of new patients coming to the women's clinic than come to the John Hunter Clinic (Table 4.6). A lot of

Table 4.6. Attendance category at women-only clinic (WOC) and John Hunter Clinic (JHC), April–October 1991

	WOC (n = 216)	JHC (n = 277)	
New patients	68 (31.5%)	43 (15%)	p < 0.001
Follow-up*	91 (42.1%)	155 (56%)	p < 0.01
Re-book†	57 (26.4%)	79 (29%)	
HIV tests	40 (19%)	26 (9%)	p < 0.01

* Attending for result or ongoing treatment.
† Re-attending with a new problem; previously attended at either JHC or WOC.

women are being referred elsewhere by health care providers; about half of our patients are referred specifically from GPs or family planning clinics. It tends to be the younger and the older age groups that are referred to the women's clinic. We also have referrals from our local children's home, the children's ward and gynaecologists. So we feel that health care workers find this clinic easier to send women to. We have also had women from the ante-natal clinic come along.

During the first year, approximately 60% of the new HIV-positive women in our unit came through the women's clinic, and the total number we have seen is about 40. We aim to integrate the HIV-positive women into our overall service with time, because they are eventually going to need both in-patient and day-care facilities, which are obviously mixed; but the women seem to find it easier to enter the service through the women's clinic.

HIV testing was initially running at 19% of all attenders, and now 25% of all the women coming through our clinic have an HIV test after counselling. We are not sure why the proportion of women being tested is so high. Certainly, a lot of women are coming specifically for an HIV test, but the staff in the clinic do their utmost to offer HIV testing, counselling and advice to all the women that are coming through. Working in the evening you are not interrupted by phone calls or messages coming through, so perhaps you can deliver a slightly more concentrated service.

Table 4.7. HIV-positive women: comparison of attendance and use of services in the women-only clinic (WOC) with the same doctor's clinic in the Kobler Centre

	Number of women (WOC)	Number of women (KC)	
Booked in for appointment	16 (100%)	14 (100%)	
Attended first appointment	14 (88%)	9 (64%)	$p < 0.05$
Attended regularly for follow-up	15 (93%)	6 (43%)	$p < 0.05$
Seen by health adviser	14 (88%)	4 (29%)	
Seen by SW/OT at clinic visit	5 (31%)	0 (0%)	
Seen by DDU team at clinic visit	1 (6%)	0 (0%)	
Lost to follow-up	1 (6%)	4 (29%)	

SW: social worker; OT: occupational therapist; DDU: drug dependency unit

Reviewing the HIV-positive women in the first six months (Table 4.7): 16 booked into the women's clinic, and 14 booked in to see me in the Kobler Centre – the dedicated HIV centre. Statistically, significantly more women turned up and continued to attend the women's clinic than the Kobler Centre, and we lost one patient to follow-up at the women's clinic, whilst we lost four in the Kobler Centre. So, it would appear that the women are morely likely to come and to return when we provide the women's clinic

Table 4.8. Riverside termination of pregnancy rate

1988 – 2564 TOPs in Riverside women
• 40% of conceptions terminated
• 35.3% performed via NHS
• Riverside TOP rate = 29.8%1000 women
• National TOP rate = 12.1%1000 women
1991
• Riverside TOP rate = 30.9%1000 women
• NW Thames TOP rate = 17.9%/1000 women
• National TOP rate = 12.2/1000 women
1993 – Chelsea and Westminster Hospital
• Capacity 1000 TOP slots per year
• Actual available for Riverside – 500 slots

TOP: Termination of pregnancy.

Table 4.9. Contraceptive use in sexually active women attending genitourinary medicine clinics

	Total	Always using contraception	Sometimes using contraception	Never using contraception
John Hunter Clinic	86	51	25	10
Charing Cross Hospital	102	75	10	17
Westminster Hospital	93	73	10	10

services.

Our family planning services – contraception, as we should be calling them – were brought on board because of a very high risk of unwanted pregnancy in our clinic attenders (Table 4.8). In 1990 we did a survey, and in the John Hunter Clinic, 41% of women (who were not trying to get pregnant) were at risk of unwanted pregnancy (Table 4.9). A year later, within the building we were in, a family planning clinic was provided – not in our clinic, but upstairs – and there was a decrease in the risk of unwanted pregnancy, but this was not statistically significant.

We all know that STDs are common in women seeking contraceptive advice. So, we provided an integrated family planning service – this is provided by staff who are trained in family planning, HIV and genitourinary medicine. In the first year, just over 100 women attended. Previous STDs were documented in half of these women. Out of 113 women, 70 terminations in pregnancy had been performed in total, and 11.5% had used 'morning after' contraception.

STD screening was attempted in all patients. We managed to screen 80% of women within three months of their first attendance at the family planning clinic. We found a significantly large number of STDs in our patients. It is also interesting that bacterial vaginosis was extremely high; these are women who were at risk of pregnancy and new data show bacterial vaginosis is a problem in pregnancy. *Chlamydia* continues to be higher than in the mixed-sex clinic, as does genital herpes – which seems to be going up and up; *Trichomonas* is now increasing.

What did we do? We changed the method of contraception in about 60% of women. Quite a number of women have gone on to depo-provera and the HIV-positive women who were attending our family planning clinic have shown interesting requests for the double contraceptive method (the double Dutch method) discussed in Chapter 2. They had previously been advised to use condoms, but they are very concerned about unwanted pregnancy. Quite a few requested depo-provera specifically to stop their periods, because they find the psychological trauma of periods is quite high. It is reminding them of their fertility and their need and want to have children. So, 16% are using a double method of contraception and this was advised by the doctor, based on their sexual history, and their STD screening and – in many cases – based also on their partner's sexual history.

However, despite this, when they arrived at the family planning clinic a number of patients were already pregnant – five in total. Three more became pregnant during the first year, and we have a conception rate of 71 per 1000 in our first year, in our family planning clinic. This has continued to be the case, and when we have looked at the follow-up of our clinic, it is very poor. So, despite providing the services on one site, only about 20% of women bothered to come back to our clinic. So, what are we going to do?

We have decided that we are not going to give up, we are going to continue to maintain the close links, continue to screen the women, continue to give them advice based on their sexual risk factors and their lifestyle. But we are going to try and improve the re-attendance rate and we are going to give them alternative family planning clinic lists, and so on. The doctors themselves are making the appointments. We are recalling patients who did not attend, and we are going to continue educating staff in the general mixed clinics and in the local family planning clinics; hoping that, wherever these women go to, they will continue to get the education and advice that they need.

What are the problems? Our biggest problem we found was with cleaners because we run the clinic at night. It is an incredibly busy clinic that goes on very late, and the cleaners get cross because they cannot clean the department. The second biggest problem is the lack of translators. We do attract women from many different countries, many of whom do not speak English, and finding translators in the day is enough of a problem, but at night it is almost impossible. The evening is a problem for some women, and particularly perhaps for those whose religion or culture does not allow them to be out alone at night.

Funding – obviously, initially, I was greatly criticised for starting this service because it is a luxury. But we are seeing more new patients and more sexually transmitted infections. It is the busiest clinic I do in the week. So I think it is very cost effective, and our purchasers are certainly supporting us at present to continue the service.

Security – we do have male security guards in the building, but we have not had to call on them.

To provide a women's only clinic you have got to have enough staff. When we started this clinic, we only had three part-time women working in the department and I ran the clinic myself; there was nobody who could do the clinic for me in the event of illness or holiday. We now have a lot more female staff and it does make it much easier.

In some ways running a women's only clinic means you are pulling your staff every way – so, it is quite difficult. But, on the whole, we feel it is successful and I have had total support from all the staff within the clinic. The male doctors certainly appreciate the clinic and refer many patients, as do the male staff in, for example, gynaecology and family planning. There certainly has not been any resentment at all by male staff.

5 Sexual health and drug use

Tim Rhodes

I am going to be presenting some findings on the sexual behaviour of drug injectors – recruited as part of an ongoing WHO funded study. I shall discuss briefly the way in which drug users perceive sexual risk in the light of everyday risks, which are part and parcel of the drug-using lifestyle. I will be making some very basic points which illustrate why drug users may not be accessing sexual health services as much as sexual health workers would like them to, and a few words about how drug users might prioritise sexual risks as less immediate and as less important than drug-related health issues.

Over the last five or six years there is a whole host of research evidence which has been pointing to changes made by drug users in their drug use and injecting behaviour. Rates of syringe sharing are still on the decline. The sharing of syringes is no longer the 'norm' within most social networks of injectors and sharing only continues under certain social circumstances and in certain social situations.

Similar changes have not been made in the sexual behaviour of most drug users and most drug injectors. We are at the point now, and have been for the last two years, of questioning (a) whether further reductions in syringe sharing can be made within social networks of injectors, and (b) whether changes in the sexual behaviour of drug users are possible. This leads us to the important question of why changes in sexual behaviour are less common and less likely among drug users and drug injectors.

Andrew Moss, a senior researcher, has termed the potential for sexual transmission among drug injectors as the 'real heterosexual epidemic'. Concerns about sexual transmission and sexual risk behaviour among injectors have been further highlighted by *The Health of the Nation* strategy – which emphasises that HIV is 'primarily a sexually transmitted disease'. Hilary Clay, a researcher, looking at drug injection in the north-west of England has said 'The sexual mediation of HIV infection is a problem which seems relatively neglected by drug workers and their clients alike.'

The study from which I will be presenting findings on the sexual behaviour of drug injectors is part of an ongoing World Health Organization/Medical Research Council (WHO/MRC) funded prevalence study, investigating HIV risk behaviour and HIV prevalence among injecting drug users in London. The study employs a multi-site sampling strategy, recruiting drug injectors in a variety of settings. Crucially, these include non-treatment based settings in the community as well as treatment based settings. A number of studies in the UK and elsewhere are showing greater numbers and greater proportions of drug injectors not receiving treatment to be HIV-positive than those who have experience of drug-related treatment. It is fundamental, then, that a study looking at HIV prevalence samples injectors from non-treatment settings as well as treatment settings in order to avoid the bias in HIV positivity found in most treatment oriented or treatment based samples.

The study employs a sampling quota of at least 50% of injectors recruited out of treatment settings and recruits approximately 500 drug injectors each year, and has done so now for four years. The findings presented here relate to year two of the study – which is 1991.

HIV prevalence is assessed through anonymous collection, with consent, of saliva. Five hundred and sixteen drug injectors were recruited in 1991; of whom 53% reported current drug treatment or help, and 27% reported never having experienced drug treatment or help in the past. Twenty-five per cent of the sample were women; mean ages were round about 30 years.

Table 5.1. Sexual activity of total sample (N=516) in the last six months

77% (396) :	sexual intercourse with opposite sex partners
3% (16) :	men sexual intercourse with another man
0 % (2) :	men sexual intercourse with men and women
80% (414) :	sexual intercourse in the last six months
20% (102) :	no sexual intercourse in the last six months

Eighty per cent (the majority) in the sample reported having sexual intercourse in the last six months. This finding is comparable to a number of other studies of drug injection in the UK – and most show proportions between 60% and 85% who report some penetrative sexual intercourse in the last six months. As shown in Table 5.1, the vast majority report sexual intercourse with opposite sex partners.

Table 5.2. Mean number of primary and casual sexual partners

Primary partners (307)	1.2 (range 1–8)
Casual partners (164)	2.8 (range 1–15)
Primary/Casual partners (80)	1.5 primary partners 3.0 casual partners
Overall number of sexual partners:	2.1 (range 1–15) *(excluding clients)*

Of those who reported penetrative sexual intercourse in the last six months 80 reported having sex with both primary and casual partners. This is approximately 16% of those who report sex with opposite sex partners. So there is a degree of overlap between those reporting sex in the last six months with both primary partners and casual partners. The proportions of those reporting penetrative sexual intercourse with clients in exchange for money or drugs is 5% of the total sample.

The mean number of sexual partners is slightly higher for those reporting sex with both primary and casual partners than for those reporting sex with only primary partners *or* casual partners in the last six months. As shown in Table 5.2, this gives an overall mean number of sexual partners of 2.1 in a six-month period. The findings from the Sexual Lifestyles survey (pilot findings) indicated a slightly lower mean number of sexual partners in the British adult population as a whole over a similar time period. The mean number of sexual partners reported by drug injectors is therefore similar if not slightly greater than that in the British adult population.

Table 5.3. Frequency of condom use with partners of the opposite sex in the last six months

Frequency	Primary* N=308	(%)	Casual† N=164	(%)	Client† N=19	(%)
Always	44	(15)	54	(33)	11	(61)
Sometimes	53	(17)	54	(33)	4	(22)
Never	206	(68)	55	(34)	3	(17)

* five missing observations, † one missing observation

The majority of drug injectors (about two-thirds) report never using condoms within their primary sexual relationships, and about a third report never using condoms with casual partners (Table 5.3). Condom use is considerably higher with clients. Once again, these reported rates of condom use are similar to those reported in the heterosexual population and in the adult population as a whole (the Sexual Lifestyle survey plus surveys in Scotland of heterosexual adults). One finding of concern is that those reporting more frequent sexual encounters were less likely to use condoms. For example, 12% of those having casual sex at least once a week always used condoms, compared with 39% of those having casual sex less than three times a month. The same trend is true of those reporting sex with primary partners. This is a concern particularly in the context of the increasingly high rate of partner change, and the mean number of sexual partners reported by injectors in the last six months.

Table 5.4. Number of drug injectors with injecting and/or non-injecting sexual partners

	Primary N=307	(%)	Casual N=164	(%)
Non-injecting	136	(44)	68	(42)
Injecting	157	(51)	48	(29)
Non-injecting and injecting	14	(5)	48	(29)

When looking at sexual mixing, Table 5.4 shows that almost half of drug injectors report having sexual intercourse with non-injecting sexual partners in the last six months. This is the key to what Andrew Moss calls 'the real heterosexual epidemic'. Also, approximately half of the primary partners of injectors are non-injectors. This is more or less the same point: sexual mixing is relatively high between injectors and non-injectors.

To summarise, firstly, the epidemiological data show that the majority of drug injectors are sexually active. This is not surprising to most of us working in sexual health services, but it is a surprise sometimes to those working within drug-related services – to those who seem to hold the popular perception that most opiate users and heroin users do not have any sexual activity. This is true to an extent, depending on duration of use and dosage. But of the heroin injectors in our study, the majority (66%) were having sexual intercourse at least once every week.

Secondly, condom use is low, but it is not lower than condom use reported in the heterosexual population as a whole. This is a key finding, because if we are looking at sexual behaviour change within social networks of drug injectors, the reasons why change is not occurring may be very similar to the reasons why such change is not occurring within heterosexual populations as a whole.

Thirdly, sexual mixing is relatively high. As already mentioned this is a cause for concern for some epidemiologists who see drug injectors as the route to the 'bridge' of transmission into the heterosexual population.

Many drug injectors and drug users are not accessing sexual health services and GUM services. When they do, or when they do access drug-related services, they tend to prioritise other things over and above sexual health. They may not see sexual risk as 'risky' as do health workers themselves. We need to look at how drug injectors prioritise 'risk'. Drug injectors are going to be less likely to change their sexual behaviour if they do not see unsafe sex as risky.

To conclude, other risks are seen as more immediate and more important to drug injectors than is sexual risk. For example, in terms of everyday lives, drug injectors are more likely to be thinking about whether or not there are risks associated with the drugs they buy and the way in which they take them. Beyond the immediate social situation in which drugs are bought and used, there are other risks associated with scoring drugs, such as violence.

6 Multicultural aspects of sexual health promotion

Shivananda Khan

I am not a health professional, but I happen to be doing community work among the South Asian, Turkish and Iranian communities. I work in a culture-specific organisation and our existence is a challenge, I believe, to all other organisations who work in generic services. I want to discuss why we have developed a very culture-specific service, particularly around sexual health. We started off with HIV and AIDS and we are now moving into the arena of other sexual health issues.

One or two of the contributions this morning refer to minority ethnic communities, but much of the data presented has not had an ethnic minority breakdown. I gather that some attempts are being made, although, for example, if you look at the drug injectors, there has been no mention of 'Are there differences between different communities?'

Another point is that we have had very little data over the course of the last few years (particularly on the HIV/AIDS issues that I am involved with) on ethnicity. There is a huge debate on how you actually find out information about ethnicity and how you monitor ethnicity. One of the things that has happened, in my perception of it, is that there is a tendency to discuss the Black communities as though they are somehow all of the same origin. For example, in the London Borough of Hackney there are something like 32 languages, and that means 32 different ways of looking at the world, because language is a way that you see the world. I have very little knowledge of the Afro-Caribbean communities or the Nigerian communities or the Ugandan communities. My expertise is from the culture that I was raised in, which is South Asian. I do not expect you to also have similar knowledge about my community as well. However, this contribution is about multiculturalism. I do not like that term because multiculturalism implies a system of integration of client services. This often results in services for Black

46

and minority communities becoming subsumed under that for the majority ethnic group, or in many instances ignored completely.

In service delivery, i.e. how you deliver the service, you have got to acknowledge the culture from which clients come. For instance, how do you translate genitourinary medicine into Punjabi? We cannot do it. We do not have the terms in our languages to talk about heterosexual or homosexual; we do not have a culture that actually has an understanding of the concept of sexuality. We do not have sexuality in our cultural frameworks. All the literature that has been produced about sexual health focuses on heterosexual, homosexual, bi-sexual. These are meaningless terms within our cultural frameworks. There are very specific reasons why. It is not that we do not do these things. Oh, yes, we have a lot of sexual fun; recreational sex is just as popular in our cultures as in any other culture. We just have a different way of talking about it and describing it. The source of our identity is not who we are as an individual but who we are as part of our family. We have to recognise that sexual health is about sex, not about figures, but about behaviour and how people practise that behaviour, and in what context they practise their behaviours.

How do you talk about sex in different cultural frameworks? Our cultures have 'invisiblised' sex. We do not have a framework to discuss sex either within the family or in a public arena. So, how should sexual health be promoted within that context?

There is a mythology, in this particular case, about the South Asian communities. There is a certain hospital in South London (which shall remain nameless) and a certain purchaser in that South London hospital (who shall also remain nameless) who said that Asians did not need any HIV and sexual health information because they are monogamous. They did not practise sex before marriage, they did not have sex outside of marriage, therefore they were perfectly safe from HIV/AIDS and sexual issues!

It raises the question as to why Asian people do not normally access GUM clinics – and Dr Pillaye has mentioned possible reasons: we have no knowledge of STDs, or we do not need to access them, or we do not know how to access them, or we go to GPs. There are data to show that we do need them, that we are just as sexually active, and take just as many sexual risks as anybody else.

Asian people cannot access GUM clinics because they cannot speak the language. And when they come into the GUM clinic, first of all they have to understand what GUM means (and it is not to do with oral health), they come in and they see images on the walls which are basically European images.

In 1992, in India, 30% of sexually active men reported an STD infection – I have argued consistently that the cultural dynamics of behaviour of our communities in this country may be very similar to the cultural dynamics of behaviour in the country of origin and we need to have some comparative data.

I want briefly to go through some of these issues that affect sexual health promotion in our communities. Although I may not be talking about Afro-Caribbean, Nigerian or Ugandan communities (and I mention those specifically, because there is a tendency to talk about African communities as one community). Africa is not one country and not one language, and the Indian subcontinent is not one country with one language, and the Caribbean is not one country with one culture – Jamaican culture is very different from Trinidadian culture – the dynamics of the issues are similar, the concerns are similar. We have an added issue over language, but the main context is the issue of racism; and I have not heard that word mentioned at this conference. The context of racism is very important when we are talking about sexual health. One of the issues that has come up with our communities is that HIV and AIDS is perceived as a white issue – it is not our issue. And that has actually been enhanced because the level of information and the type of imagery used to promote sexual health services are primarily in English or, have images from a Eurocentric viewpoint. Even the attempts to translate information have proved somewhat disastrous. For example 'anal sex' has been translated as 'entry through the back door', and 'oral sex' as 'verbal sex'. But even our communities are at fault, too. I have read a leaflet produced by a Black organisation in the north of England where Bengalis were classified as racist in the translation. The real term was 'racially' but translated into 'racist'. There is no direct equivalent in translations and most people do not seem to understand that you have to develop a whole contextualised translation if you are going to get effective information.

The perception of the service providers (I mentioned the south London hospital) is that we are safe, passive, quiet, and obedient. Similar passions are aroused by Afro-Caribbean and African cultures, where concepts about sexuality and sexual behaviour abound.

How many of you know anything about our cultures, our histories, our dynamics? For instance, how many of you recognise that for various Asian cultures, marriage is relatively compulsory? In a study that I did among 1200 Asian men who have sex with men, 90% were married. Not out of choice, but because of community duty. Consequently you cannot define those men as bisexual because their main sexual partner, another man, was outside their marriage. Because our identity is with the family and because marriage is a necessary duty, our perceptions of self are different. Marriage is about children.

Another significant difference between our various cultures is the issue of shame and guilt. Some religions actually enhance the sense of personal guilt. In our cultures, the controlling factor is the issue of public shame. When an issue such as sexual behaviour, an STD infection, HIV, or AIDS becomes visible, what that produces is a culture of shame. This means that most people in our communities would find it very difficult to talk publicly about the issue, or go to a public clinic about the issue, or be visible in any particular way. Shame is what controls our behaviour. This means that we have an issue of public space and private space. What we say publicly is not necessarily what we do privately. It does not mean that we are schizophrenic, it just means that we live in two different worlds. We have different concepts of our relationships, and that is often ignored. It leads to denial and invisibility, which is why there seems to be very little evidence – public evidence – about attending clinics, about sexual behaviours or about HIV rates.

There are differences between first, second and third generation Asians in overlays and complexities. There are differences between the different language groups – Punjabi, Hindi, Urdu, Bengali. For instance, the Bengali that most Bangladeshis speak is Sylheti which is not a written language. We assume that everybody can read – and read in their own language as well – and that is not necessarily true. South Asian women have less access to the written form of the language than the men. The men may control access to information; when a leaflet comes through the door, it is a husband or the elder male that picks up the leaflet and then decides whether the wife and the female children should see that leaflet. So you have to reconstruct how you deliver your services and how you promote your services, and the only way you can do that is to consult with those people in our communities who have that knowledge and who are capable and able to do that sort of work with you. In this contracting culture, you have to contract in. So if the government wishes to attain its targets, this has to be recognised, and likewise for the funders, providers and purchasers.

To summarise – we have to acknowledge the different psycho-social structures around behaviours and identities in different cultures. If we do not, we are going to miss those communities altogether. We have to build this acknowledgement into appropriate education and awareness programmes. Also I would urge you to be careful that you understand the difference between the word 'appropriate' and the word 'sensitive'. I have seen a sensitive HIV prevention video which did not talk about sex, which is the main route of transmission in our community, so you cannot avoid it. It was sensitive to the needs of the community but it was not appropriate. We have to acknowledge the power of shame, dishonour and denial within our communities in the delivery of services, because these are our controlling factors.

We have to recognise the different histories that exist. In my country I learned all about the British Raj and the Indian Mutiny of 1857. In India, we talk about the First War of Independence, in England we talk about the Indian Mutiny! Two different ways of seeing the same event; two different psycho-social profiles that come out of the perception of that event. Each culture will look at the world differently. We have also to recognise differences in language, terminology and imagery, especially over social health.

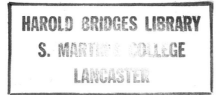

HAROLD BRIDGES LIBRARY
S. MARTIN'S COLLEGE
LANCASTER

7 Sexuality awareness for genitourinary medicine professionals

Jef Jones

In presenting this contribution I tried to think about who we are at this conference, this gathering of sexual health educators, genitourologists, researchers, gynaecologists, and I could not quite come up with a polite collective noun for us. There is a politically correct euphemism for prostitutes which I think precisely defines who we are – 'workers in the sex industry'.

What is sexuality and what does it mean? One of the immediate definitions of sexuality is that it is something that only gay men and lesbians and kind-of bisexuals possess. I have been invited to seminars and workshops about sexuality, and when I have got there, I have found that what people wanted to hear about was what it is like to be a lesbian or a gay man. So, one limited definition of sexuality is that it is gay men and lesbians who have it and maybe bisexuals have a bit of it. What is quite interesting, is that it is something that Black people also happen to have.

Sexuality is also very obviously bound up with our gender, and obviously the genders of the people to whom we may be sexually attracted. There is another politically correct euphemism that is used in the States to refer to lesbians, gay men and bisexuals, which is 'persons of orientation'. As a person of orientation myself, I am delighted to be credited with the knowledge – with some kind of sense – that I know where I am going. I know in which direction I am going, I am delighted to have that credited to me.

Sexuality is also. bound up with what we do. It is bound up with the actual sexual practices that we are involved in. It may also be bound up with the sexual practices that we would like to be involved in, but have not yet had the opportunity. It may also be our sexual notion of ourselves and maybe bound up with sexual practices which we would never want to be involved with, and are actively repulsed by.

Obviously our sexual notion of ourselves is also bound up with things which may have been done to us which we did not wish to happen; things into which we were coerced or manipulated. And, perhaps less immediately cruel than sexual abuse, I think we have all nevertheless experienced some damage or some hurt to the sexual sense of ourselves. Whether we are persons of orientation or not, we have all received, from childhood, negative messages. It is wrong to masturbate. Women should be passive. Men should perform. Now, most of us here will be aware of many of those other messages – and some of them are related to racial identity. There is a whole industry of destructive lies which affect and damage us all.

Equally, whether we ascribe to it or not, we have a national sexual identity in Britain. Sexuality is a source of cultural fascination, and a subject of moments of comic and tragic national theatre. Events become headlines news when they are subject to the glare of our national cultural relationship with sexuality – whether we actually credit that or not, that is what happens in our dominant culture. And that relationship with sexuality seems, to me, to be made up of equal parts of cruelty, fascination and delighted disgust.

Sexuality may, or may not be, one of the most important things about us. We may feel that other things define us more importantly – our religion, our community, our culture, our race, our profession, our economic status, our HIV status, our gender. These may all be more important to us as ways of thinking about ourselves than our sexuality. But what I would remind us of, is that all of those experiences and activities may also help us to compose our sexual sense of ourselves. So, all of those aspects of our lives feed into how we think of ourselves sexually.

Sexuality is a powerful and intimate way of thinking about ourselves, and a way of thinking about ourselves in relation to other people. It is an internal and intense story that we tell ourselves. Our sexuality is, in all kinds of ways, like our genitals. It is mundane, we carry it around with us, it is like a person or a mobile phone – we get it out sometimes, put it away at other times. It is part of the background apparatus of our lives. But, like our sexual organs, it can provide us with the most astonishing experiences of tenderness, of passion, of excitement and of human contact. But, also like our sexual organs, it can provide us with the most distressing experiences of isolation, shame, guilt and physical pain.

As workers in the sex industry we feel that none of this applies to us, all of that is only true of our clients and our patients. We only treat our patients and our clients less than excellently when we pay less than excellent attention to ourselves.

The task of education, of diagnosis, or treatment and of care certainly requires of us – intellectually and ethnically – that we maintain an objective and uninvolved perspective. It is vital that we are able to listen calmly and clearly to the people that we are working with. I am not disputing that. But I do want to remind us that objectivity is only useful as a tool of compassion, of healing and of enablement. In so much medical training and in so much medical practice – and I am referring here to the way we socially produce the medical persona – the way that we socially manufacture medical personnel; in that process, objectivity becomes a glamorous goal in itself and it can become effectively a way of distancing oneself from the people one is working with.

So what then occupies that gap, when we have established that distance? Whether we like it or not, we are all carriers of our culture's peculiar prejudices and erotic power systems. And, through our relationships with our clients and our patients, we can transmit our own hurts, fears and unspoken anxieties.

Where staff at all levels – and this includes directors, senior consultants and purchasers – are given the encouragement, the resources, the time and the skills, in those clinics where that happens, another tool which sits alongside objectivity becomes available. That tool for compassion and healing is nothing more complicated really than shared humanity. In the clinics where staff are encouraged to go through that process in training, consultancy, support and supervision, those become true sexual health centres; where patients are not just equally treated, but where their sexuality is dignified and celebrated.

8 Contact tracing and partner notification

Elspeth Gould

There are many diverse views on what partner notification is, and on its utility.

The World Health Organization (WHO) states that partner notification is that spectrum of public health activities in which sexual partners (or in the case of HIV – needle sharing partners) of people with STDs are notified of their contact, counselled on their exposure and offered appropriate services. The person with STD might do this him- or herself (i.e. patient referral)[1] or a health-care worker, such as a health adviser, might notify partners (i.e. provider referral)[2].

This system is well established in many parts of the world, Britain included. What was originally called contact tracing started at Newcastle General Hospital 50 years ago[3]. Throughout that time, partner notification has been neither directive nor coercive, it is a co-operative venture with the person with STD. It must be carried out with a great deal of confidentiality; that of the person with the infection, and of the partner who *may* have been in contact with infection. We owe at least as much confidentiality to the contact as to the index person.

I would suggest that partner notification is concerned with both primary and secondary prevention. Identifying people with previously unrecognised infection and providing treatment is secondary prevention. Other contributors have provided graphic reminders of the damage and grief that may result, for example, from untreated *Chlamydia* infection, and with such bacterial infection we can offer cure. Viral infection cannot be so neatly sorted out. However, we can work with people with bacterial and viral infection, again in a co-operative manner, to help them to protect themselves from further infection and to protect others from new infection. This is primary prevention. Partners can be given information and the time to talk and think about the choices they have to protect themselves. This gives individuals who are sexually active, and who have already been in contact with STD, the opportunity to discuss how they can protect themselves in future.

Back in 1980 the Health Education Council produced *The Handbook on Contact*

Tracing in Sexually Transmitted Diseases. Already it looks dated, as are some of the illustrations – it is hard to identify with the people hanging round in discos looking for 'Lisa with the red hair' to come in. But there is quite a lot of good stuff in that handbook, and the five-stage contact tracing interview is part of that. It reminds us that, unless you have a good relationship with the index patient, you will get nowhere. Part of building that relationship is talking about the present infection, how it was or was not acquired, what the treatment consists of, and how this person can be safer in the future. This helps the person who is already using the services, and forms the basis for the partner notification. Thus partner notification promotes the sexual health of the index person.

And the partner who is notified, whether by the patient or by the health care worker, has the chance to make informed choices about attending a clinic, and being screened for infections. It may be that the contact partner wants to be tested solely for the infection that the index patient has, but the gregarious nature of STDs should be borne in mind and full screening offered. Where bacterial infection is found and cured this necessarily protects future partners – primary infection. The partner who attends a clinic, whether infection is found or not, has the chance to discuss prevention of infection in the future.

Having looked at the theory, does partner notification work? There are different ways to view 'success' in this endeavour. One is to record the number of contacts who may be traceable, the number of them who are known to have attended for examination, and of those who were examined how they got their infection(s). Table 8.1 gives examples of these figures for our clinic for 1991 (this is the last year for which these figures are available). One notable feature is the number of 'other infections' that are found.

Table 8.1. Outcome of partner notification (NGH GUM, 1991)*

---

801 with NSGI named 693 partners, of whom
285 are known to have been examined:
85 had no treatment, 53 were given epidemiological Rx,
109 had NSGI, 106 other infections were treated.

---

353 ♀ with NSGI named 246 ♂ partners, of whom
119 are known to have been examined:
12 had no treatment, 29 were given epidemiological Rx,
61 had NSGI, 24 other infections were treated.

---

88 ♂ with GC named 64 ♀ partners, of whom
35 are known to have been examined:
4 had no treatment, 4 were given epidemiological Rx,
23 had GC, 26 other infections were treated.

---

607 ♂ with warts named 485 ♀ partners, of whom
146 are known to have examined:
106 had no treatment,
22 had warts, 57 other infections were treated.

---

* Newcastle General Hospital GUM clinic.
NSGI: non-specific genital infection; GC: gonorrhoea.

Another way of looking at the outcome of partner notification is to check the proportion of people attending the clinic with a particular infection who attended as a result of partner notification. Table 8.2 gives examples from our clinic for 1993, generated by computer. Nearly a third of our female patients with *Chlamydia* attended solely because of partner notification. These are women who might have developed pelvic inflammatory disease had they not been informed that they were at risk of infection. Of the male patients who had had sex with men, gonorrhoea was found in 28.9% of those attending as contacts. Rectal and pharyngeal gonorrhoea are frequently asymptomatic, so this should not be surprising.

Table 8.2. Outcomes of partner notification (NGH GUM,1993)*

Of 1678 partners named, 605 (36%) are known to have been examined
Of 304 ♀ patients with *Chlamydia*, at least 99 (32.6%) attended because of partner notification
Of 45 gay/bisexual ♂ patients with GC, at least 13 (29.9%) attended because of partner notification
Of 604 ♂ patients with warts, 81 (13.4%) attended because of partner notification
Of 502 ♀ patients with warts, 57 (11.4%) attended because of partner notification

* Newcastle General Hospital GUM clinic.
GC: gonorrhoea.

Patient referral is far more common than provider referral for all infections in our clinic, but we have only quantified this for HIV infection. We looked back over a seven-year period and found that of the 80 partners attending as a result of partner notification, 79 were tested. Twenty-five (31.6%) of these were seropositive. This was 21.9% of our newly diagnosed case-load. Seventy-five attended following patient referral and five as a result of provider referral[4].

Partner notification has demonstrated its contribution towards sexual health promotion in genitourinary medicine.

Definitions of partner notification, patient referral and provider referral (WHO, 1991)

Partner notification – the spectrum of public health activities in which sexual partners of individuals with STD and HIV infection are notified, counselled on their exposure and offered services. (Needle sharing partners of people with HIV would also be notified.)

Patient referral – The approach whereby an infected patient is encouraged to notify partner(s) of their possible infection without the direct involvement of health care providers.

Provider referral – The approach whereby . . . health-care workers notify a patient's partner(s). The infected patient provides information on partner(s) to a health worker, who then confidentially traces and notifies the partner(s) directly.

References

1. WHO (1990). *Prevention of Sexual Transmission of Human Immundeficiency Virus.* WHO, AIDS Series 6. WHO, Geneva.
2. WHO (1991). *Management of Patients with Sexually Transmitted Diseases.* WHO Technical Report Series 810. WHO, Geneva.
3. Gould, E. M. (1993). Tynesides schemes for the control of veneral disease. In *Medicine in Northumbria: Essays in the History of Medicine,* (eds) D. Gardiner-Medwin, A. Hargreaves, and E. Lazenby. The Pybus Society, Newcastle-upon-Tyne.
4. Parttman, R. S. and Gould, E. M. (1993). Partner notification for HIV infection in the United Kingdom: A look back on seven years' experience in Newcastle-upon-Tyne. *Genitourinary Medicine,* **69,** 94–7.

9 A service user's perspective

Mohammed Rajabali

This contribution is about my own experiences and talking to clients at Cruisaid. I have collated the points most frequently raised by various people about their experiences at different clinics round London.

At the first visit to an STD clinic there is a tremendous amount of anxiety and fear engendered, and surprising as it must seem these days, still a lot of shame associated with it. The question of actually going into a clinic and feeling unclean is quite a common reaction. There is a different type of atmosphere between an STD clinic and an HIV clinic. In an STD clinic, especially if the client is male and under-age, he is not only afraid of the fact that what he is practising is illegal, he has no idea how he is going to be treated. I am talking now about the gay male perspective, because I really do not know how either a woman or a straight person would feel, but from a gay point of view, for a young gay going into an STD clinic and suddenly realising that what he has been doing is actually illegal – he may wonder: What will happen? Will the doctor say anything? Will he be condemned? Will he be reported? There is a lot of fear of the unknown.

These days, the fear has been compounded by the fact that catching an STD equates with unsafe sex, and all the associated anxieties of AIDS, of being HIV-positive. The attitude of the nurses, doctors and social workers is extremely important on the first visit, as is the treatment of the current condition and also the question of whether the client should have a test or not.

In the HIV clinic the same fears apply, but the attitude of the doctors and nurses is markedly different.

Should there be an appointment system run at these clinics and what are the pros and cons?

Firstly, the pros. I am in favour of appointments as long as they are actually kept. Everyone needs to take time off work to actually go to a clinic and it is often difficult to explain to colleagues where they are actually going. The only way they can do it is plead sick and take the day off, and then hope that everything will be done in one day and they do not have to take another day off. With an appointment system, such visits can be planned and there will be the least amount of stress to the client.

Secondly, the cons. Against that, you have clients who may discover something and want to know something fast and cannot get an appointment to see the doctor for several days. Or clients may not turn up – and that happens – or appointments are running late. However, no one actually tells the clients why appointments are running late, and it would be such a small thing to do. But these are all minor irritations which can be overcome.

One question which came up frequently was, should there be separate STD clinics and HIV clinics. There were mixed feelings about this. When you actually go to an HIV clinic, you are suddenly different. Also there is a stigma attached to going to an HIV clinic, because it is like going to an STD clinic, especially if the clinics themselves are located quite close to each other. Location does matter a lot, especially if they are for example, located on different floors. That sort of problem could be easily solved.

Again the appointment system comes in here at the HIV clinic, because people really are much more stressed. They often want a much longer time between clients. Personally, I must say that, given this fact, I am very much in favour of appointments in HIV clinics – and I think it actually does work on the HIV side.

Another point which comes up is the changing of doctors. This can be quite traumatic. In an STD clinic it may not matter so much, because it may be something you have just caught and this may be the first time; it may be cured and you go home. But if you are in an HIV clinic you will be seeing the doctor over a long period of time and it is a question of building up a relationship. I know of clients who are on their third doctor in 18 months and quite often they only find out they have a new doctor when they arrive for their appointment and find that the doctor they thought they were to see is no longer there. It would be preferable if they could be told by the doctor that he/she is leaving and so break it to the clients gently. This comment especially is quite relevant. I understand that doctors have careers to pursue. However, on the user side (especially on the HIV side), clients have become much more demanding than they ever have been in the past.

The art of listening to patients was also seen as important – i.e. the discussion of patients' lifestyle, the alternative therapies available which could complement the drugs, etc. A lot of the time, the solution still seems to be to just apply medicine or to give drugs that are known to cure. This often appears to be the first solution, rather than a presentation of choices. People should be presented with some choices, they should be actually given the opportunity either to take drugs or not. There have been cases on both sides – I know clinics vary (some clinics are better, some doctors are better), but, in some places the only choice a client has been given is 'Here is some medicine to take' and that is it. I think, in a lot of cases it would be nicer, or more relevant actually, if people's lifestyles were discussed – i.e. how they actually live. What is relevant here is to discuss the question that there should be some suggestions of changing of people's lifestyles. Some clients are still behaving in instances of long nights, drug abuse and a lot of alcohol. The question of discussing the client's lifestyle, explaining to him how things could change if he also changed his lifestyle, if there actually is a complementary solution to do with the way he actually lives, the way the drugs will affect him, the way he can lower stress. The clients must be presented with these choices.

Someone who has been told that he has AIDS and realises he may not have very long to live, will be in total shock. He needs much more consideration than would probably be given at an STD clinic.

The question of drug trials was often raised. How are people actually being recruited for drug trials? Is pressure being applied? Do clients feel emotionally blackmailed into trying them if particular hospitals are trying to reach their quota of people they want to have for drug trials? Are alternative therapies actually ever discussed with clients? I know it is a lot to ask of doctors to spend more time with their clients but, especially for HIV-related patients, these clients may feel they have only a very short period of time to live; which may not always be true. The initial prospect, however, is that they always feel that they may not have much time, and a lot more understanding is required for them.

The patient–doctor relationship is also an aspect raised, namely, how is the client going to obtain, for example, benefit claims. This is perhaps going much further than people actually expect of a doctor, but this is the type of question that comes up – how willing are doctors to sign for sick notes for disability payments? The same rules do not apply from clinic to clinic. Sometimes a doctor's relationship with his/her client governs this. Also, it may be an easy way for a doctor to sign a note under pressure from the client, but it will not always be a good thing for a client to stop working on getting a positive diagnosis. Can he actually cope with the thought of just having so much time on his hands? Is the job always so stressful? These are things which need to be discussed with the client as well.

Another question that came up was about patients becoming in-patients at the clinic they attend. What sort of liaison is there between in-patient records and GUM clinics? There has always been the question of bureaucracy. Again, do the records leave the GUM clinic and actually go to the in-patients' side? These may be just fears expressed by clients, because they do not actually know what the situation is. Everything may actually work, but there is always anecdotal evidence – 'Oh well, we did not hear about this' or 'The doctor did not know about my allergy to this drug, which he could have found out if he had read my notes from the GUM clinic'.

As far as women's GUM clinics are concerned, the only person I could canvass for any kind of opinion was our social worker. Her only comment was that there has always been pleading from her women clients on the question of crèche facilities. And I have no idea what the planning is there. Wherever there have been crèche facilities, there have been good reports from their women clients.

When providing a service, how far should you actually go? What role has the client's doctor now taken on – is he going to be a confessor, a financial adviser, does he also advise on how to claim benefits, does he have to state what benefits are on offer. Do you provide counselling for the client, the partner, the family? Just how far do you go? It is very, very difficult these days to discuss these sorts of things.

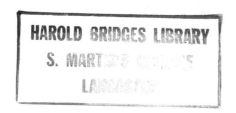
HAROLD BRIDGES LIBRARY
S. MART...
LANCAS...

10 The perspective of a clinical nurse – services offered by genitourinary medicine clinics

Veronica Poon

The role and responsibility of a clinical nurse specialist in the GUM clinic varies from clinic to clinic.

As a clinical nurse specialist (CNS) in the Florey Unit, there are two distinctive roles:

- To manage and teach the nursing staff in the unit.
- To liaise and participate in educational programmes on sexually transmitted diseases, including HIV and AIDS, for health-care professionals and external agencies in hospital, and in the community (health promotion/education)

Three major groups of nurses will be discussed in this contribution.

Nursing trainees – Project 2000 nurses

The GUM department is not included in the curriculum for 'traditional' nurse training. Many qualified nurses have little or no knowledge about the working of a GUM clinic.

The new style of nurse training – Project 2000 – places greater emphasis on health promotion and ill health prevention. Their curriculum includes an input from the GUM department about its services, and a brief description of sexually transmitted diseases, treatment and prevention.

The aims of the lecture are to:

- promote self-awareness;
- recognise what are sexually transmitted diseases;
- know how to use, or recommend others to use the services of a GUM clinic.

It is hoped they will stimulate an interest in some of these nurses to specialise in GUM and thus help future recruitment.

Practice nurses

This group of trained nurses is on the increase and many of them are practitioners in their own right. They carry out primary and secondary health education and health promotion in the GP surgeries; they hold screening clinics like well man and well woman clinics, family planning clinics, etc.; and they are in daily contact with their patients.

My aim is to provide information to this group of nurses about the services of a GUM department so that:

- They have a better understanding of the service.
- They encourage clients to use its services.
- They explain to their clients the facilities available.

How was I approached?

Organisers of different courses attended mostly by practice nurses, invited me to give talks to their delegates about the GUM department. Many of those who attend often request further sessions about sexually transmitted diseases. Others recommend their peers to invite me to their place of work to dicuss their needs. I have also compiled a booklet for them to use as a reference at their workplace.

Community school-nurses

This group of nurses working in the community is my latest contact.

Many of them are running drop-in clinics at their secondary schools and have found them a valuable use of their time. It was emphasised that these drop-ins were a move to a better means of meeting the health needs of the secondary school age pupils.

The topics discussed at these drop-in clinics were monitored and the most common subjects discussed were:

- Relationships (as in boyfriend and girlfriend).
- Sex and sexual health.
- Contraception.

These community nurses felt that they were lacking in confidence in the area of sexual health and contraception and expressed a need for study days with input from family planning and GUM. These are being organised.

The aims of the study are to:

- improve and update knowledge;
- be more confident and comfortable to discuss topics with their pupils;
- use resources (leaflets) available.

The Government's White Paper *The Health of the Nation* has set out general objectives to reduce the incidence of HIV and other sexually transmitted diseases, and to reduce the number of unwanted pregnancies. This inspired a group of community school-nurses and health visitors to form a committee 'Teenage Pregnancy', with input from family planning, GUM and health promotion departments.

The general objectives of *The Health of the Nation* – HIV/AIDs and sexual health were used as guidelines by the committee to organise:

- A roadshow – stall/stand in a shopping mall.
- A drop-in centre (one evening a week) staffed by various agencies.

I would like to conclude with a quotation from *The Health of the Nation*: 'The Health of the Nation* is a strategy for health, not ill health, or even health care. The strategy emphasises the need for active partnerships – healthy alliances – between the many organisations and individuals to work together to improve health'. A clinical nurse specialist in a GUM clinic has an important role in the healthy alliances that promote sexual health.

A purchaser's perspective

Rochelle Bloch and Anthony Worth

Purchasing sexual health promotion – Rochelle Bloch

The two questions which come to my mind, and probably most purchasers' minds are: 'Why should you purchase sexual health promotion?' and then, 'How?' So, very briefly, this is going to be an overview of why, looking at *The Health of the Nation*, epidemiology, local activity and some sort of cost benefit perspective to purchasers (Table 11.1), and, how to look at contract specifications and some work on quality standards and the role of health promotion. Anthony Worth will expand on that area.

Table 11.1. Purchasing sexual health promotion

Why?
The Health of the Nation
Epidemiology
Local activity
Cost/benefit
How?
Contract specification
Quality standards
Role of health promotion

Looking at *The Health of the Nation* you could, with a cynical view actually say, well, we could achieve the national gonorrhoea target without really doing much different from what we are currently doing (Table 11.2). We could achieve it without particularly doing any more work on sexual health promotion with gay men or other priority groups. Perhaps not so much in the district I represent, but nationally I think that you could excuse people for taking a fairly relaxed view of achieving this particular target.

Table 11.2. *The Health of the Nation*

- Gonorrhoea target
- ?Work with gay men or other priority groups

HIV/AIDS
- High local incidence
- High local GUM clinic attendance

Other STDs
- Changing patterns
- Range of organisms
- Serious sequelae
- Many asymptomatic

For us in Ealing, Hammersmith and Hounslow, we have to look at the issue of HIV and AIDS – we have a very high local incidence (we are in the region with the highest incidence and prevalence in Britain). I know that in Ealing, Hammersmith and Hounslow there have probably been about 600 reported AIDS cases to date and that 50% of them are in the Borough of Hammersmith and Fulham. We know that about 800 people are known to Hammersmith and Fulham Social Services – either symptomatic or asymptomatic with HIV. So, it is a real purchasing issue for us.

We know that, locally within the region (i.e. within central London), we have a very high GUM clinic attendance – much higher than the rest of the country. And that is important – it shows that we have a high incidence of STDs, and that is relevant to our local population.

Table 11.3. **Some long-term sequelae of sexually transmitted diseases**

Pelvic inflammatory disease
Infertility
Cervical cancer
Liver cancer
Major systems disease
Neonatal disease
AIDS
Psychosexual problems
Chronic urogenital problems

Other STDs are also important. There is a changing pattern of STDs and there is a range of organisms involved. There are a number of serious sequelae, and many are asymptomatic. We think it is quite important that people come to GUM clinics with asymptomatic diseases because this can prevent secondary infection and long-term consequences (Table 11.3). So, we do not think that this is a waste of money (Table 11.4) and perhaps it is something that those who are purchasing sexual health in other districts should think about, because it is the mark of a good quality service. While we know that the rate of gonorrhoea is decreasing for both females and males, other STDs are increasing. The gonorrhoea target, therefore, is somewhat misleading and not very helpful when looking at promoting sexual health.

Table 11.4. *Chlamydia trachomatis* – a suitable case for population-based treatment?

Estimated direct cost associated with sequelae of untreated *Chlamydia trachomatis* infection

Condition	£
Acute pelvic inflammatory disease	
Inpatient	1000
Outpatient	90
Cervicitis	50
Infertility	2000
Chronic pain	500
Ectopic pregnancy	2000
Neonatal pneumonia	400
Neonatal conjunctivitis	30

Table 11.5. *Chlamydia trachomatis* – a suitable case for population-based treatment?

Background
- Intracellular parasite
- Sexual and intrapartum transmission
- Multiple immunological types
- Largely asymptomatic
- Treatment cheap and effective
- Variety of associated diseases:
    - male non-gonoccal urethritis, urethritis and epidydimitis
    - female cervicitis, pelvic inflammatory disease
    - neonatal conjunctivitis and pneumonia

For the long-term consequences of STDs, I think it is important for purchasers to realise that they are wide ranging and could have major, costly outcomes (both physically and emotionally) for the people involved. And this is something that I would be saying to my health authority and why we have to continue purchasing sexual health promotion and sexual health services.

It might be useful to look at the work done on *Chlamydia* in our region (Table 11.5). This is an asymptomatic infection in a lot of people, who might not even know they are carrying it. We know that the long-term sequelae that can occur with untreated *Chlamydia* infection can be, for example, pelvic inflammatory disease (PID), with consequent infertility, ectopic pregnancy and risks to obstetric and perinatal events.

Rochelle Bloch and Anthony Worth

These factors from a purchaser's perspective are important because they involve costs and the costs of treating these different sorts of episodes can be quite high, especially for ectopic pregnancies, infertility and acute PID.

These people are unlikely to have been identified as carrying *Chlamydia*, because the services are not geared to picking that up. So, actually encouraging people to come in to GUM clinics with asymptomatic infections for sexual health screening is probably a very good tactic on the purchaser's behalf. That is one example that I have some figures for (Table 11.6) – it is not the only one by any means.

Table 11.6. *Chlamydia trachomatis* – a suitable case for population-based treatment?

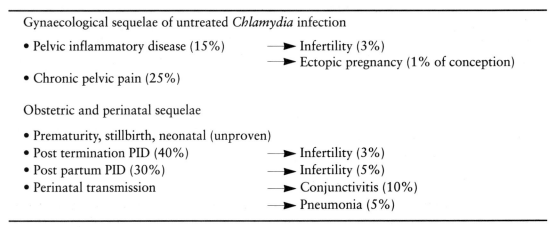

As purchasers, if we look at our local population needs (Table 11.7), we have a range of issues about trying to determine these accurately. Information is insufficient as we do not have proper breakdowns of our local population, partly because most services are open access. So, it is difficult to tell which of the local population is accessing services in which local clinic. At the moment we do not have the breakdown of where people are coming from. I do not think this is an argument against open access services, but it is useful for all purchasers to know where their residents are accessing services so they can look at either improving their local services or to maintain current arrangements. So, borough-based data are currently unavailable – and that is something we need to look at.

Table 11.7. Local population needs

- Current information insufficient
- Open access services
- Borough-based data unavailable
- GUM clinic is only contact with NHS for some clients
- Large sexually active population (national survey)

Need to develop systems for defining the population-based epidemiology of sexually transmitted diseases
- HIV, gonorrhoea, *Chlamydia*

The GUM clinic is, for some, the only contact they have with health services. We need, therefore, to make sure that these clinics address other health needs, for example contraception and cervical cytology, and to make sure that people get the services they need and not that they are just being treated for the presenting condition.

My district has a large sexually active population. We know that from the recent national sexual behaviour survey – particularly in inner London. And we have to make sure the services are there. In order to develop services we need to have proper systems for defining the population-based epidemiology of STDs – particularly HIV, gonorrhoea and *Chlamydia*. And that is something, as purchasers, we need to work very hard on. I think it would be difficult to have a strategy for sexual health services without having that information, or, to make any major changes. We do not really know what we need to be providing. We know that there is a demand, we know there is a need, we know that it is cost-effective, and we need to continue doing it. All we can do at present, is work on some guiding principles for what sort of services we want to provide and what sort of things should be in the contracts.

Table 11.8. Guiding principles

Diagnosis and treatment of sexually transmitted diseases is primary prevention.
Sexual health promotion through risk reduction and clinical service.

Provision should be the objective of sexual health interventions.

Respect for consumer choice, empowerment and the rights of the individual must underpin all services, including the right of an individual to make informed choices about their sexual and drug taking behaviour.

There are three major principles, and these are ones that have been developed from the work of our regional focus groups (Table 11.8).

- The diagnosis and treatment of STDs is primary prevention – by treating a disease in a person presenting at a clinic, you are preventing them transmitting that infection to their next sexual partner. This is very important – probably more than any other service – that primary prevention, diagnosis and treatment are linked together.
- Sexual health promotion should be the prime concern of any sexual health intervention, as well as looking at risk reduction and clinical service provision. Sexual health promotion is part of the service – it is not an add-on. One question I was asked was, 'Is there a trade-off between GUM services and sexual health promotion?' Well, I do not see that there is a trade-off, they are one and the same. It is part of the quality service when providing sexual health through a GUM clinic service – you should be offering sexual health promotion as part of that. I do not think there is any either/or in that at all.
- Consumer choice. I think it is worth reiterating one of the principles we have learned through HIV – and it has to be maintained throughout – is that respect for consumer choice has to be part and parcel of the service we offer. Respect for their choice of sexual behaviour, or drug taking behaviour, or whatever. That is important. That has to be within the service that we offer; it is part of the quality; it is what we should be buying.

What, therefore, should be in a GUM contract (Table 11.9) that will help to ensure we can meet those principles and that we can provide a good quality service? (I have

Table 11.9. Key elements of genitourinary medicine contracts

- Open access and confidential
- Friendly and welcoming

- Easily accessed:
  – evening clinic
  – signposted

- Well publicised

- Targeting those not accessing services:
  – drug users
  – Black and minority ethnic communities

- Collaborate with other sectors/services:
  – family planning
  – schools and colleges

- Offer routine hepatitis B screening and immunisation

- Have colposcopy policy:
  – criteria for colposcopy
  – links with primary care screening

- Provide regular demographic and geographic activity data
  for sexually transmitted diseases and HIV/AIDS, including KC60 returns

- Provide training in sexual health promotion and
  communication skills for all staff

not included HIV testing in this, as in our authority we have separate service specifications – one for HIV and one for GUM services; because in some of our clinics they are separate.) Obviously all that we know about pre- and post-test counselling would also be included. A lot of this is basic stuff from the Monks Report of the working group to examine workloads in genitourinary medicine clinics (DHSS 1988 MC/7737a) (Table 11.9).

- Services should be open access and confidential. They need to be friendly and welcoming. They need to be easily accessed – you need to look at whether you want evening clinics, or a weekend clinic once a week (and that depends on the pattern of demand from the clients – local needs as assessed). You need to look at signposting and where the clinic is – whether it is on a hospital site, whether it is at the front of the site, or whatever, so people can find it. It needs to be well publicised. Also it needs to look at targeting those who are not accessing services appropriately. In our district we are interested in actually working more with drug users and people from Black and minority ethnic communities who we know under-use current GUM services.

- The GUM service needs to collaborate with other sectors and services; it needs to look at links between family planning and GUM – for example, whether or not you have a family planning clinic at the GUM clinic once a week. Whether you have good referral patterns, whether you offer post-coital contraception as part of the GUM service, all these issues needs to be worked out. And, of course, what are the links with schools and colleges and local sexual health education. It is important that a team approach is established. And that, again, I see as part of the contract – part of what we are buying from a GUM service.

- We would like to have routine hepatitis B screening and immunisation offered through GUM services. This is a preventable, asymptomatic, STD. Obviously, we need to look at what that means in terms of costs – especially in our area of London.

- Another area of interest is colposcopy. It seems to me that while there is a need for colposcopy within GUM, there is a lot of overlap between gynaecological and family planning services, and it might be useful to look at what criteria are used for colposcopy and how to link these with the primary care screening programme. This will be something we shall be looking at as a new thing for GUM services in 1994.

- More local data collection and training of health professionals is required. As already mentioned we must get better data. I think that traditional arguments about confidentiality under the Venereal Diseases Act should not obstruct this process. We need aggregate, borough-based data in order to look at how we plan services, and also to look at changes in local epidemiology. We need to work with clinics to develop systems. I know that this is an area which has been looked at as a regional issue in North West Thames.

- We need to ensure that training in sexual health promotion and communication in sexual health matters is available for all staff – doctors, nurses, reception staff, counsellors, health advisers, and other.

The role of health promotion in service development support – Anthony Worth

I shall discuss briefly, what both Rochelle and myself see as the role of health promotion in service development support – particularly in the area of GUM. My presentation is divided into four areas (Table 11.10).

- The role of HIV infection in challenging clinical practice.
- The changing face of health promotion services.
- Support in setting and maintaining quality standards.
- Potential problems regarding perceptions of such a collaboration between the purchaser and provider of health promotion.

Table 11.10. The role of health promotion service development support

---

- The role of HIV infection in challenging clinical practice
- The changing face of health promotion services
- Support in setting and maintaining quality standards
- Potential problems – perceptions of purchasers/provider collaboration over quality issues

---

The role of HIV infection in challenging clinical practice

It is really important to recognise that HIV has focused people in terms of their clinical practice, particularly over sexual health promotion and in the direct provision of sexual health services (Table 11.11).

Table 11.11. The role of HIV infection in challenging clinical practice

---

- Confidentiality
- Proactive access provision for different communities
  e.g. lesbians, gay men, Black and ethnic communities, refugees, people with learning difficulties, people with mobility problems
- Collaboration with other sectors/services (especially voluntary organisations) – sexual health teams, school and college teams
- Provision of greater choice in terms of services and resources

---

While confidentiality has always been recognised as an important issue by GUM services, it has become an issue of even greater importance with the advent of HIV and AIDS. HIV infection has also encouraged people to be more proactive in providing access for different communities, rather than providing a standard generic service that is supposed to meet the needs of all communities. Within the diversity of communities to be targeted are lesbians, gay men, Black and minority ethnic communities, refugees, people with learning difficulties and people with mobility problems. That list is not exhaustive or exclusive, just a beginning, looking at the needs of the more obvious groups. GUM clinics do need to examine access issues for *all* groups.

Collaboration with other sectors has been focused with the advent of HIV infection. Of significant importance is the voluntary sector, often overlooked, but nevertheless an important reservoir of great expertise, having in many cases pioneered many policies and practices. Naturally, statutory sector teams and agencies (e.g. sexual health teams) should not be overlooked.

An issue for consideration is the provision of greater choice, both in terms of services and resources attached to those services. It is simply not good enough to remove the clinic's one condom from its locked drawer, wave it about a bit with the immortal words, 'You are using one of these, aren't you?', and then slam it back in the drawer. Clients need open access to resources which they recognise, feel comfortable with and are suitable for their particular needs. The same must be said for services.

The changing face of health promotion services

It should be recognised that, nationally, there is probably no standard model of health promotion agency, as we are in the midst of reform (Table 11.12). In West London Health Promotion Agency (Ealing, Hammersmith and Hounslow) we are moving into the sphere of advice and consultancy; provider support, and liaison and network management, promoting links between statutory services and voluntary organisations where they do not already exist. Many GUM services have already shown themselves to be proactive in their voluntary sector relationships.

Table 11.12. The changing face of health promotion services

Move towards
- Advice and consultancy
- Provider support
- Liaison services
- Advocacy
- Purchasing advice
- Contract management

Away from
- Resource provision (solely)
- Traditional prescriptive approach

West London Health Promotion Agency (WLHPA) has moved away from the traditional function solely of resource provision. I think it is important that we maintain a resource provision service, but we should be equally proactive in supporting the development of appropriate resources for different communities. We are also moving away from the old traditional prescriptive approach to health education (in this case, HIV prevention).

Support in setting and maintaining quality standards

The ways in which we as an agency intend to set, support and maintain quality standards is through the medium of collaborative planning with GUM services to set up monitoring systems (Table 11.13). The message is 'doing things with services' rather than 'doing things to services'. For example we are able to advise on what quality benchmarks might be most appropriate when setting up monitoring systems. We are also able to provide access to existing models of quality standard setting as well as to other professionals versed in the required skills. It is important to set structures which

Table 11.13. Support in setting and maintaining quality standards

- Collaborative planning with GUM services – setting up monitoring systems
- Advice on quality 'benchmarks'
- Provision of access to models of quality standard setting/other professionals
- Setting a structure – meeting purchasing requirements
- Examples of standard setting/client consultation

meet service users requirements as well as purchasing requirements. These are important in that the following questions should be able to be answered within the structure:

- How do we know that we are actually providing quality services?
- Do we know that we are being effective?
- Are we providing the most relevant service for the community groups within our locality and can those groups access them?

When looking at the GUM based standard, the same model applies, regardless of the issue to which the standard statement applies. Structural reviews are especially important when setting standards. In this example, the standard statement is:

- The health professional will offer contact tracing advice for all individuals diagnosed with syphilis, gonorrhoea and *Chlamydia*.

The structure for this standard statement is:

- A quiet room is needed to ensure privacy. Confidentiality is paramount. The discussion should be free from prejudice and at level of understanding acceptable to the patient.

The *outcome* of this standard will be:

- All individuals, where appropriate, will be offered contact tracing.

Patient/client questionnaires are, I feel, essential tools in the evaluation of quality standards. Questionnaires should be preceded by an explanatory note and a statement regarding confidentiality of respondents. Examples of questions that will prove useful are:

- Were you able to ask questions at any time during your visit?
- Were all your questions answered?
- Were facilities available for you to speak to the (GUM) staff in your preferred language?
- What is your preferred language?

(Naturally, it should be recognised that if a client's first language is not English then they may have difficulty in answering such a questionnaire! Access to good reliable interpreters is essential. Failing that, questionnaires should be available in the main languages spoken in the locality.)

- Were you able to choose the doctor that you saw?

- Did you know the name of the doctor who looked after you?
- Was your physical examination carried out by a nurse of your choice?
- Did you feel safe?
- Were you comfortable?
- Did you have to wait long?

Potential problems regarding perceptions of collaboration between purchaser and provider over health promotion

To conclude, it should be recognised that no collaboration happens without problems or potential problems (Table 11.14). I think that we have been very proactive in WLHPA in working through some of those problems. The main one being that the health promotion agency has been perceived as punitively monitoring on behalf of the purchasers.

Table 11.14. Potential problems – Perceptions of purchasers/provider collaboration over quality issues

---

- Health promotion may be perceived as promoting 'punitive' monitoring methods on behalf of the purchaser.
- The role of health promotion (generally) may not be fully understood (need for PR exercise).
- GUM services providers will be less likely to accept support over quality issues if initial training and support is not provided.

GUM services will be less likely to accept support with regard to quality issues if training and support is not provided. It simply is not on to go into a GUM service and tell the service that one is going to set up monitoring systems. Approached in such a way, a GUM service is likely to be less co-operative.

Support should be planned and should provide the initial support and back-up required to monitor quality standards and help all concerned towards a common goal.

12 A clinical director's perspective

Dr George Kinghorn

I am conscious that many at this conference are already converted to the idea that opportunistic sexual health promotion should be carried out in a GUM clinic.

My contribution will generally be in agreement with the other contributors especially those from Ealing, Hammersmith and Hounslow. However, not all purchasers share their views.

In the real world, there are two major problems which have to be overcome. Firstly, additional resources are necessary if effective sexual health promotion is to be carried out. Secondly, there are persisting attitudinal problems amongst some providers and purchasers.

There are clear epidemiological associations between STDs, unwanted pregnancy, anogenital cancers, infertility, neonatal infections, and HIV/AIDS. What can also cripple people is the psycho-social/psycho-sexual morbidity which often accompanies this wide spectrum of disease. Both the acquisition of a sex related disorder and the unconfirmed perception that one may have acquired such a disorder can be injurious to normal well-being. When we focus upon the management of one of these conditions, it is important that our concern should extend to all related health problems. It has, in my experience, often been extremely difficult to get health care professionals who are involved in HIV/AIDS prevention and treatment to understand the association with other STDs and sexual health problems. I consider HIV/AIDS testing centres that do not also focus upon other STDs as a potential disaster which may permit a preventable and/or treatable disease to harm their clients.

Peter Greenhouse talked in the first morning session (Chapter 3) about the problems of young teenagers. We have recognised for many years that there is an association, especially in girls, between broken homes, sexual abuse, running away, so-called promiscuity, unsafe sexual practices, prostitution and drug use. These young people may access the health service at a variety of points. Many access hospital services on a

Friday night, having taken an overdose. But they are discharged the following morning without anyone considering the associated issues. Young people who lack the love and security provided by a caring, family environment will often seek that love elsewhere and leave themselves vulnerable to the abuse which, thereafter, results in this recognised chain of events. GUM services need to recognise these problems and aim to intervene where possible.

Service objectives for GUM clinics are the prevention, treatment and control of STDs, HIV/AIDS and associated genital tract conditions. To achieve those objectives, we need to promote

- Early patient presentation – encouraging them to present to clinics when they perceive themselves to have been at-risk of acquiring an infection, rather than delaying until symptoms have appeared.
- Prompt and accurate diagnosis by efficient and comprehensive microbiological facilities.
- Efficient treatment regimes, with appropriate clinical and microbiological follow-up to ensure infections are cured.
- Patient education, support and counselling, in a non-jugemental fashion.
- The co-operation of patients in seeking the attendance of sexual partners in order to prevent re-infections.

What special opportunities has GUM for sexual health promotion? The acquisition of STDs sensitises patients. The majority of individuals believe that 'It's never going to happen to me', and therefore take little note of educational messages. Those who acquire an STD develop a more realistic state of risk perception, and the educational messages take on a new personal relevance.

In our outreach work, GUM health workers have credibility with target groups. By their clinical experience and up-to-date knowledge of the subjects they are discussing they can have enhanced impact. Personal contact with at-risk individuals always promotes clinic attendance. Other aspects of our outreach activities, such as performing provider referral during contact tracing procedures, have already been addressed by previous contributors. However, all of these services have an associated cost.

I would like to illustrate this by outlining some of the work my health advisers are involved with in the provision of health care for prostitutes. I am a long-standing believer in providing health education at the place of work – whether this is on the street or in the sauna. This work is time-consuming, and resource intensive in terms of health adviser time, free condoms and hepatitis B vaccine. However, there are considerable cost-benefits from improving the health of sex industry workers and reducing their role in the local transmission of STD. One strategy which has stimulated regular clinic attendance is the issuing of dated 'freedom from infection' certificates which then confer advantages upon sex workers in their negotiations with the managers of saunas.

It is important to identify and develop partnerships with women who can act as peer educators. They can help promote healthy attitudes and practices among young girls newly working in the industry, especially those who may be using prostitution to finance a drug habit.

Financing of GUM services is within block contracts which allows open access to any patient, irrespective of their district of residence. There are no waiting lists. My service agreement is based upon historical workload; funding relates to the number of new patients and their total clinic attendances. In almost all of the acute hospital services, funding is based upon the numbers of ill patients seen; there is little or no reward for disease prevention. If the basis for funding was changed in favour of disease prevention, then attitudes to health promotion among service providers would surely change. The high costs of management for HIV/AIDS patients is but one reason why this should change.

In most contracts for GUM services there is an absence of case-mix data – that is, there has been little attempt so far to differentiate between patients with differing types of illness, which have widely differing associated costs. This means that patients with HIV/AIDS whose care is staggeringly expensive, are often funded in a similar way to those with uncomplicated genital infections.

Even when a GUM service has been successful in obtaining additional resources for HIV/AIDS patients, then rapidly increasing numbers can effectively deplete the resources which are available for other routine activities. In the USA, and in some London centres, there have been adverse effects upon basic aspects of the service, such as contact tracing for STDs, as a consequence of high HIV/AIDS workloads. Many centres have had to abandon outreach work in this vital area. This is a false and unwise economy, for the more untreated STDs there are within the communities, the more HIV transmission will ensue. Therefore, it seems that the present funding mechanism will reward bad clinical practice and lead to more infected patients.

Another funding problem, which particularly affects major conurbations where there are higher incidences of STD and HIV/AIDS, relates to the policy of equalising funding between teaching and non-teaching health districts. This has led to an absence of development funding in many provincial cities. My purchasers, who have been obliged to reduce expenditure on acute services by £20 million, will not kindly receive requests for any service development, no matter how justifiable, in these circumstances.

What we are now proposing are for fewer patients throughout the clinic, because of the longer consultation times required for effective health promotion, at potentially higher cost. If clinic hours are to be extended, for example, to accommodate the special needs of particular groups, then the additional staff involved will have to be paid. Medications, hepatitis B vaccine and condoms all cost money which has to be found. If staff are to be effective in their wider educational roles, then funding for their training will have to be sought. Our clinic services will be more expensive, and if they are effective, will be treating fewer patients. They are likely to be viewed as being less effective by purchasers as the cost per patient rises. Are those who are 'strapped for cash' prepared to pay for an unproven service, albeit of higher quality, at the present time?

Our outreach activities will also have a funding requirement, some of which was outlined earlier. In addition, we should not forget the essential funding for monitoring and evaluating these activities.

Let me be constructive about the potential solutions in the current financial climate. There is scope for redeployment of existing resources. For some conditions we need to reduce follow-up rates. We certainly need to develop shared care protocols, to develop better liaison and collaboration with general practitioners and other community health care professionals. We would be greatly assisted in our proposals if we could provide definitive proof of the value of sexual health services. Sceptical purchasers will not pay for those proposals, which although based upon common sense and 'gut reaction', have not been proven to be effective by appropriate research.

Research and evaluation of new initiatives must go hand-in-hand with all new service developments. This alone will convince sceptical purchasers and providers when they are confronted with a passionate interest in health promotion.

Although I have been a little sceptical and cynical in this contribution, I believe that the most important question to which we should seek a solution is not 'Can we afford it?' but rather 'Can we afford not to?'